THE
Tresillian
Sleep Book

Expert advice on how to help your baby
to sleep – from Australia's most
trusted parent support organisation

ABC
Books

The ABC 'Wave' device is a trademark of the
Australian Broadcasting Corporation and is used
under licence by HarperCollins*Publishers* Australia.

First published in Australia in 2018
by HarperCollinsPublishers Australia Pty Limited
ABN 36 009 913 517
harpercollins.com.au

HarperCollins*Publishers*
Level 13, 201 Elizabeth Street, Sydney, NSW 2000, Australia
Unit D1, 63 Apollo Drive, Rosedale, Auckland 0632, New Zealand
A 53, Sector 57, Noida, UP, India
1 London Bridge Street, London, SE1 9GF, United Kingdom
Bay Adelaide Centre, East Tower, 22 Adelaide Street West, 41st Floor,
    Toronto, Ontario, M5H 4E3, Canada
195 Broadway, New York, NY 10007

A catalogue record for this book is available
from the National Library of Australia

ISBN: 978 0 7333 3914 1 (paperback)
ISBN: 978 1 4607 0945 0 (ebook : epub)

Cover design by Michelle Mackintosh
Cover image by amana images/ Getty Images
Internal images by Shutterstock.com
Typeset in Minion Pro by Kirby Jones
Printed and bound in Australia by McPherson's Printing Group
The papers used by HarperCollins in the manufacture of this book are a natural, recyclable
product made from wood grown in sustainable plantation forests. The fibre source and
manufacturing processes meet recognised international environmental standards, and carry
certification.

About Tresillian

Established in 1918, Tresillian is Australia's largest early parenting organisation providing family-focused care for thousands of families each year. With services rapidly expanding to reach more metropolitan and regional areas, Tresillian helps parents gain confidence in their roles as mums and dads and provides evidence-based education and support around breastfeeding, infant sleep, settling and nutrition to maximise each family's wellbeing.

> Need advice? Contact Tresillian's Parent Helpline on 1300 272 736 or go online for advice at tresillian.org.au

About the author

Fran Chavasse is a registered general nurse, registered midwife and is a child and family health nurse. Fran's specialty is infant mental health and she has as a Master of Mental Health (Infancy). Fran is currently doing a PhD; her research examines the nurse and mother's adult attachment and how it affects their working alliance.

Fran has worked in child and family health nursing for more than 35 years. Her primary expertise is in the first 5 years of life, and she has also worked with children through primary school and into adolescence. She has worked in a wide range of child and family health services, including extended health home visiting, mother and baby residential units, clinical nurse consultancy and nursing management. As senior nurse educator for Tresillian, Fran regularly provides a range of infant mental health workshops for child and family health nurses, allied health professionals and childcare workers.

About the editors

Deborah Stockton is a registered general nurse, registered midwife and child and family health nurse. Debbie's focus has been the provision of care and support for families in the early years of their child's life, working across a range of child and family health services in metropolitan and rural locations including community nursing, mother and baby residential units, telephone helpline, clinical nurse consultancy, nursing management, education and research. She is currently undertaking PhD research which aims to enhance access to services for families in rural communities. Debbie works at Tresillian as the Operational Nurse Manager – Regional Services.

Nicola Brown is a registered nurse with extensive experience in children's nursing in health care services, staff development and the higher education sector. She has contributed to professional texts and journal publications on acute and chronic illness in childhood and adolescence and families, and professional development for nurses. Nicola's areas of research interest include parents' management of their child's illnesses and promoting health for their children. She is currently a PhD candidate, undertaking a study to explore family-based interventions to promote a smoke-free home. Nicola works at Tresillian as Nurse Manager of the Professional Practice and Innovation Centre.

Acknowledgements

I would like to thank the people who have provided me with support, encouragement and contributions for this book.

I am very grateful to Debbie Stockton, Tresillian Operational Nurse Manager – Regional Services, for reading, editing crazy sentences, providing comments and changes to content and suggesting improvements for each chapter of the book as it was written. Debbie has been with me all the way and her help has been invaluable.

I would like to thank Nikki Brown, Nurse Manager Professional Practice and Innovation Centre, for her final editing, adding her paediatric expertise and providing me with the time and support to write the book.

I would also like to thank Caitlin Wright, who interviewed all the mothers and wrote up their stories for the book.

I also received wonderful support from Ann Paton, Tresillian's Public Affairs and Marketing Manager, who managed the production of the book and guided me through the process.

Thank you to both Troy Trgetaric, Tresillian Director of Corporate Services, and Robert Mills, CEO of Tresillian, who gave me the opportunity to write this book and made sure I had the time and space to do it. I have really enjoyed it.

Finally, I need to acknowledge the contributions of my colleague Denise Findlay at NCAST Programs at the University of Washington, Seattle, USA. NCAST Programs have made a great addition to my comprehension of the language of infants and they are used extensively at Tresillian Family Care Centres. Parts of this book have been informed by the education gained by my Instructor-level training in the NCAST Parent–Child Interaction Feeding and Teaching Scales, and some of the terminology and information about non-verbal cues contained in Chapter 6 are gratefully sourced from NCAST Programs.

Fran Chavasse

CONTENTS

CHAPTER 1

How sleep works

First things first, let's look at what sleep is and how it works.

Does your baby just know how to sleep when she's born? Does she sleep like you or is there something different about the way your baby sleeps? And who made up that phrase 'sleeping like a baby' and what does it mean?

Probably, as far as you're concerned, 'sleeping like a baby' is one of the most ridiculous things anyone has ever said. Whatever that phrase originally meant doesn't really matter, because this book is going to explain to you what 'sleeping like a baby' really means.

Your baby's sleep is part of her physical development, just like learning to walk and talk. Sleep is linked to many important parts of her development, such as early brain maturation, learning and memory, social and emotional development and physical health. The maturing of your baby's sleeping and waking cycles is one of her most important developmental tasks.

You might be reading this and saying, 'Yeah, yeah – just get to the part where you tell me how to teach my baby to sleep all night.' That information is included in these pages, but before reading any further, here are two important questions to ask yourself:

1. Could someone teach you to sleep longer than you need to?
2. Could someone teach you to sleep when you don't need to?

Whatever your sleep-deprived brain just whispered then about 'being able to sleep forever' or that persistent thought that you would have no problem being taught to go to sleep anytime, those two questions don't have simple answers. No one can make you sleep longer than what your brain tells your body it needs to sleep, and no one can make you sleep when your brain isn't ready to sleep.

Except for when your baby is unwell, I'm sure you have already figured out she doesn't sleep longer than she needs to, and that you can't make her go to sleep. That's why you're reading this book.

This will be disappointing news, but there is no simple, magical formula that will teach your baby to sleep. Sleep is complex, and it follows a normal developmental course similar to the way your baby develops the ability to walk and talk. Sleep is controlled by the body's natural rhythms, with the master control centre deep in your baby's brain.

In this first chapter, we'll look at new and different information about sleep that might help you understand how it begins to develop and what you can do to help your baby's sleep development. There's also information about your baby's 24-hour body clock, which is her first important sleep rhythm to establish. This helps with the development of her later sleep rhythms. The next chapter will cover the second rhythm to develop: how she begins to sleep longer through the night.

Circadian rhythms

One important factor about sleep that's often not talked about but plays a big role in your baby's sleep is our natural circadian rhythms. These are the 24-hour day–night rhythms that involve physical, emotional and social tasks.

Healthy sleep is linked to the timing of these particular internal daily rhythms:

- the cycles of light and dark, which synchronise the sleep–wake rhythms
- body temperature
- the hormone melatonin, which induces sleep.

And to these external daily rhythms you can add:

- feeding
- social contact
- activity patterns.

In the early period after birth, your baby's internal biological clock is maturing its functions. Each of these rhythms takes time to develop over the first few months of her life.

You might ask what's so important about them. Research has found that parents who help their baby synchronise her day–night rhythm to a normal daytime–night-time 24-hour clock soon after birth have a much more enjoyable relationship with their baby. So, it's useful to understand how you can synchronise your baby's daily biological and external rhythms. Here's how you can do it.

Your baby's day–night rhythm

Firstly, think about humans throughout evolution. We have adapted to a world of waking with the sunrise and going to sleep when the sun goes down. In the natural darkness, the moon, stars and some sort of fire at night were the only sources of light. Your baby's biological clock needs to be set to that traditional day and night rhythm – not a modern one with lots of artificial light.

For the first four weeks of her life, your baby doesn't follow a normal day and night pattern – she doesn't wake up with the sun or go to sleep when it gets dark. But you can help your baby begin to develop this natural day and night pattern right from the start of her life.

During these first four weeks, your baby sleeps and feeds every 2 to 4 hours, day and night. At about 4 weeks of age, your baby becomes more wakeful during the day, especially just before or after sunrise. In fact, your baby's biological rhythm of sustaining awake periods during the day comes 'online' before her ability to sustain longer periods of sleep during the night. So, bright light will make your baby more awake, but darkness won't always stimulate sleep – that's important to remember.

It can seem that your baby has the ability to stay awake, especially if you keep her in a bright, stimulating environment – which makes sense when you think about it. You are probably just the same. It's important for you to know this, because it helps you to understand why it's sometimes difficult for very young babies to go to sleep.

After your baby is 2 months old, she will probably wake at sunrise – anywhere between 4.30 am and 7 am – and you may have difficulty resettling her at this time of day. This also happens at the end of the day, around sundown, anywhere from 4 pm to 7 pm. This is often the time when your baby will be very grumpy and cry a lot (see Chapter 5: Why your baby cries).

What does all this mean and how can it help you? Well, you can organise your baby's routines to help her internal and external rhythms adjust to day and night. And the way to help your baby coordinate her day–night rhythm to the 24-hour day is to expose her to natural sources of light and dark so her rhythms develop naturally and on time.

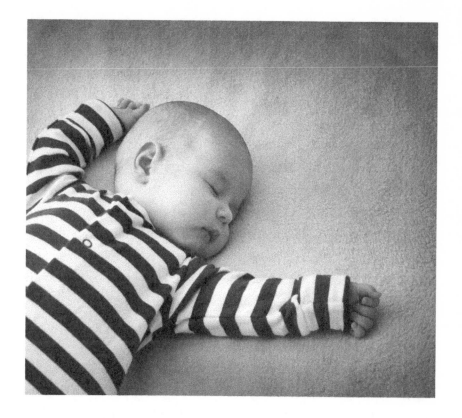

The role of light

First off, your baby needs exposure to natural bright daylight in the morning and early afternoon. It's common today for us to spend much more time indoors than outside. This means your baby will get lower levels of natural daytime light, which can affect her daytime activity and alertness.

On the flipside, we've extended daylight by the use of artificial lights. Exposure to artificial light at night can delay the development of your baby's natural circadian rhythms, plus it extends the length of your baby's day much longer than she can cope with. And with the extra light usually comes extra socialising from the family or visitors, and additional visual stimulation from the TV or other electronic devices. Your baby's feeding rhythms may be disrupted too, and she may be fed when she's not hungry because she is fussing and tired. When she's fussing because of overstimulation and tiredness, it might be hard to see whether she's ready for a feed or sleep. You might find it harder to read her non-verbal communications (see Chapter 6: How your baby communicates).

The type of light you use at night also affects your baby's rhythms. Artificial light doesn't compensate for daylight as you might imagine. Researchers have been studying the types of light that affect our sleep. Up until recently, people used old-fashioned light bulbs that gave out a yellow light. Now fluorescent lights and short-wave blue lights are increasingly used in the home, which seems to affect circadian rhythms and sleep, especially in the evening. Televisions, computers, tablets, smartphones and handheld game consoles have lights with blue wavelengths that are very stimulating and can keep babies awake much longer into the night.

How melatonin and body temperature work

Melatonin is a hormone that induces sleep and is produced during the night. For the first six weeks of her life, your baby's melatonin is beginning to establish its rhythm. It can take just a little longer to come 'online' than the day–night rhythm. By about 10 to 12 weeks, her melatonin is establishing its day–night rhythm.

Melatonin rises at night and reaches a peak in the early morning hours, when your baby is sleeping. Your baby's body temperature is also linked to melatonin. As sleep approaches at night, body temperature drops and melatonin will start to rise. Lower body temperature seems to induce drowsiness and then sleep.

Because melatonin production is connected to the day–night cycle, you can help establish your baby's melatonin rhythm through the way you care for her. You can help her natural rise in melatonin throughout the night, with the accompanying drop in body temperature, by ensuring a predictable period of night-time and lights out.

Help establish your baby's day–night rhythm

- **Get more natural daylight outside.** Take your baby for short walks in her pram out in the sunshine, especially if your house doesn't have much natural light. It's important to follow the SunSafe guidelines for protecting your baby's skin (see cancer.org.au/preventing-cancer/sun-protection/). Make sure to keep your baby out of direct sunlight as much as possible when UV levels are 3 and above. Also, sunscreen isn't recommended if your baby is less than 6 months old. Dress her in light clothing and a hat to cover her up.

- **Get more natural daylight in the house.** Keep your curtains open and let the daylight in so both you and your baby have increased exposure to natural daylight. If your house is dark, turn the lights on if possible, especially during the first eight to 10 weeks. Greater exposures to light in the day and natural dark at night will help both of you to sleep better.

- **Have a consistent bedtime.** Put in place a predictable and flexible bedtime routine each evening with a predictable lights-out time (see Chapter 4). Your baby's bedtime doesn't have to be exactly at sundown – just a regular bedtime when your baby enjoys prolonged quiet and darkness each night. Short periods of dim light for feeding won't be a problem.

- **Keep lights dimmed.** Having bright lights on at night will interfere with synchronising your baby's melatonin to her circadian rhythm and reduce the amount her body produces.

- **You also need a good night's sleep.** You will benefit from a predictable period of lights-out time and decrease in blue-light exposure 2 to 3 hours before bedtime. This down time will help your circadian sleep–wake rhythm.

Breastmilk is melatonin-rich at night. Research suggests breastmilk contains levels of melatonin that mirror the normal day–night pattern. Absent during the day, melatonim levels start to rise as the sun sets and peak between 2 am and 6 am. If you're breastfeeding during the night, your baby will get the added benefit of melatonin in your milk, which may also help her sleep.

When you help your baby establish a day–night rhythm, she will adjust to socialising and feeding more during the day and this, in turn, starts the process of her longer night-time sleeps. With your help, by 10 to 12 weeks your baby will have longer wake periods and be very sociable during the day, extend the periods between her feeds and begin to sleep a little more at night (see Chapter 7: Working on your sleep problems: Birth to 6 months).

Once again, though, you need to keep your baby away from those pesky bright lights at night. That means establishing a bedtime routine where your baby has a 'lights-out time'. The bright lights at night interfere with the way your baby's melatonin synchronises to the day and night. If she is exposed to too much artificial light for too long into the evening, this may reduce the amount of melatonin her body produces, so it's important to try and keep lights dim. There's research to suggest that lights with a long wavelength – yellow and red lights – may be less stimulating for both you and your baby. So, when you need to feed her, change nappies and attend to her, try a night-light or hall light with a yellow-ish light. At least, then, you won't be bumbling around in the dark.

Remember that your breastmilk contains melatonin and it follows a day–night pattern. Just like your baby, you need low light for a rise in melatonin or it will also be delayed. If you're breastfeeding, this could mean you and your baby's melatonin won't be synchronised during the night – your melatonin may rise much later in the night and early morning than hers.

When you maintain a predictable bedtime routine and reduce the use of blue-light exposure before bedtime, this will help with your breastmilk melatonin levels as well and keep you and your baby biologically synchronised.

But why do you need to be biologically synchronised? Because it helps with her social and emotional development. All aspects of her development are connected to each other.

Another interesting thing to consider is the time of day when you express milk to give your baby. You have no melatonin in your daytime milk, so if you are going to offer your baby expressed milk at night, try to give milk that you've expressed during the night. Your night-time expressed milk has melatonin, and by giving her that at night you are providing melatonin when she needs it for a good sleep.

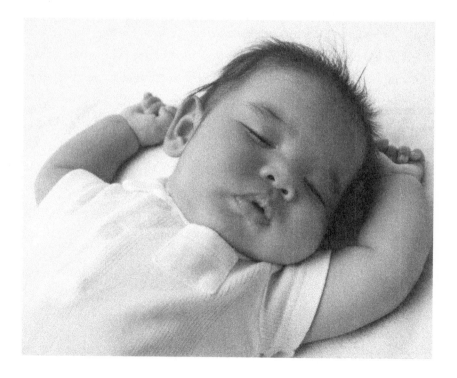

You might be saying by now 'All this is a bit much! I have a life too!' And this is a totally understandable sentiment from you; as if you aren't sleep-deprived enough. The main thing for you to know is that this information regarding circadian rhythms is an important piece of the sleep puzzle that can help you make sense of how your baby's sleep develops. There are some important ideas to take from this section that may comfort you:

- Your baby's sleep develops slowly and in stages.
- You have ways to help your baby.
- Any information you have can be modified to suit your family's needs.

You never know if it will work unless you try, and you may also benefit from rearranging your day–night routines along with your baby's. Both mood and the early phases of sleep are thought to be affected by fluorescent and blue light. Although at first you will experience lots of disruption to your sleep because your baby is going to wake you up during the night, reducing artificial light may help your day–night rhythms to improve and, when your baby eventually sleeps longer, your sleep will quickly improve as well.

Being in sync with your baby, especially during the first three months, really helps for the development of long-term sleep patterns.

External daily rhythms

This might seem like an obvious thing to say, but light is the cause of your baby's activity. People are not nocturnal and have always been active during the day, and so is your baby. That's why bright light keeps your baby awake. Sometimes this simple thing gets a bit mixed up with babies and people will give you lots of conflicting information. Basically, remember that your baby is just like you, with the same human requirements – just in baby format.

Feeding, socialising and activity patterns

Daytime is the time to socialise together, enjoy social feeding times, learn about your baby's activity patterns, learn who she is as a little individual and delight in her. Night-time is sleeping time, quiet feeding time and no socialising time. She is learning to distinguish day and night.

At 6 weeks, your baby is awake more during the day and sleeping more at night. At first, your baby will sleep in short sleep cycles of 40 to 50 minutes. And she may sometimes sleep longer than that, which means she can join some sleep cycles together. You may have heard of that.

Joining sleep cycles together is a different sleep rhythm to the day–night circadian rhythm. This rhythm takes longer to develop and will be explained more fully in Chapter 2: Sleeping longer through the night.

Your newborn baby's sleep, feeding and activity times are all unpredictable as they are 'free-running' around the 24-hour clock; that is, she feeds and sleeps at any time during the day and night. This can be tiring and stressful if you're not prepared for it, for at least the first four to six weeks. These are normal feelings and experiences during the early months.

Throughout the first four to six weeks, you help to coordinate your baby's day–night rhythms by establishing a regular resting, feeding and activity routine. At the same time, you are synchronising yourself with your baby by responding understandingly when she needs you, trying to learn what she needs and working with her to get her into day–night patterns. Let's look at ways to do that.

Establish a flexible daytime routine. Your routine doesn't need to run like clockwork. Not many people live their lives hour-by-hour on a clock! If you think about getting to work every day at the same time, even that can get tedious. Everyone lives by routines, and some are more flexible than others.

Think about your life before you had your baby. When you had to go to work, your routine might have been pretty tight sometimes – maybe you were under the pressure of timeframes or deadlines – but at weekends you had greater choice of how to spend your time. You still had a routine, but it was most likely a bit different. Maybe you got out of bed around the same time each weekend (later, because you didn't have kids), had breakfast, lunch and dinner when you were hungry, but your meals were probably still around the same time as your normal weekday. Just a bit more flexible but possibly within about an hour of the usual time you do something. Or maybe your weekend routine was the same as other weekends – socialising, cleaning but flexible. Do you see what routines are? Everyone has routines; some people like more rigid routines than others – but most routines are still fairly flexible, familiar and predictable. Routines make people feel safe and comfortable.

Similarly, routines for babies generally run on a flexible timeline, but they are familiar, predictable and responsive to your baby's needs – pretty much like your own. Your baby will also want to feed when she's hungry and not by the clock. So, feeding times will always be 'around about' a certain time (see Chapter 6: How your baby communicates). Most feeding and sleeping routines seem to run flexibly about an hour either way. That means if your baby fed at 2 pm and you think your baby may feed again in 3 hours at 5 pm, don't be surprised if she feeds anywhere between 4 pm and 6 pm. As she gets older, her feeding routine will become more regular, but it will never be exactly 3 hours or 4 hours apart. People just don't eat like that – or most don't.

Make feeding sociable. When she's little, your baby will tell you she's hungry by crying, fussing, trying to eat her hands and turning towards you eagerly. She will look like she's all curled up with her little hands tucked under her chin or reaching out to you. She'll take your breast or bottle eagerly and seem happy. Usually, she'll suck loudly and gulp her milk.

If the feed is during the day, this is the best time to socialise and let her know that daytime is social time. Feeding is when your baby is mostly awake, particularly during the first three months, and it's especially important that you use this time to socialise with her.

Think about when you have meals with your family. What do you do when you share a meal? What do you talk about with your family and friends? The socialising part of a meal is probably what you focus on far more than the food. You enjoy the food but what's even better is talking about your day or, if it's a romantic dinner, focusing on each other. When you think about sharing a meal, we often sit opposite so we can see each other's face and eyes.

The socialising, love and affection is what your baby needs far more than just the food. This is what helps her brain to grow. She needs her meals with you to be a social time in daylight. She also needs to be awake to feed properly, so this is an upbeat time for her. This is when she will be learning about the world and about affection from you.

The sort of socialising she will like is cuddling close when you're giving her milk feeds – she will be happy with whatever feeding method you use, whether breast or bottle. Tell her that the feeling in her tummy is hunger and that she's drinking milk. That seems kind of obvious, but she doesn't know it yet. You can tell her you're going for a walk later or she's got beautiful brown eyes. Sing to her, tell her stories, smile at her

– she'll enjoy any social interaction. In fact, she'll enjoy that more than whatever you're feeding her. When you talk to her, smile at her, stroke her and cuddle her.

If you're worried you will interrupt her feeding by doing all that, the trick is to just go slowly. When she's enjoying her sucking and drinking happily, let her just feed and wait until she has a break and looks at you. She'll tell you when she wants to have a chat. When she stops to have a break, talk to her. Again, think about when you're having a meal with someone. You stop talking to eat, enjoy your food and then join in the conversation again. You also wait for other people to finish their food. Your baby has the same needs as you.

During the night, feeding is just for nutrition so there's no upbeat socialising. But that doesn't mean you act like a robot. You might have been told not to make eye contact with your baby at night. This isn't true, and not making eye contact will distress her. Your baby gets all her information through her senses: vision, hearing, touch, taste and smell. She needs to make eye contact with you for love and reassurance. Imagine if you wanted to make eye contact with someone you loved and they just kept looking away without speaking to you. That would be confusing and distressing.

> When you provide calm, rhythmic, repetitious and soothing behaviours, you're more likely to keep your baby calm.

Therefore, still make eye contact during night feeds and anytime you're attending to your baby at night. Use soothing, rhythmic touch and speak in a quiet and soothing tone. Keep the lights dim to maintain a clear division of day and night. What you're trying to do is regulate your baby's day–night rhythms so she begins to set her biological and social day–night rhythms.

When you provide calm, rhythmic, repetitious and soothing behaviours, you're more likely to keep your baby calm. At night, keep the feeding and lights-on time as short as you can. This will be hard at first, but the more you try to keep a consistent rhythm, the better you can move towards synchronising your baby's day–night rhythms.

Selecting a pram

The best type of pram for your baby is one that faces you, so she can see your face all the time and gain constant reassurance. Imagine being in a pram at knee level, facing people and animals coming at you really fast! Your baby needs to face you.

It's popular to cover your baby's pram with a light cloth when she sleeps to block out stimulation but this isn't absolutely necessary. Your baby needs to be able to see your face to gain emotional support and reassurance, especially in loud, stimulating places. Your face, gentle touch and soothing voice will help to reduce stimulation far more than covering her with a cloth. You may decide to use a light cover to help reduce sunlight and keep insects off your baby when you're in the open air. More importantly, though, if you are using a cloth to cover the pram, make sure there's really good airflow into the pram so the inside is a safe and comfortable temperature – this will avoid your baby overheating.

Car safety

Whenever you're travelling by car, make sure you have the correct baby capsule or car seat for her age and ensure it is fitted properly on the back seat. Babies from birth to 6 months are safest in a rear-facing restraint seat, which offers the best protection, even once she's 6 months old and over. If your baby is too long (or tall) for a rear-facing child restraint seat, and she's more than 6 months old, you can put her in a front-facing seat with a built-in six-point harness, also placed on the back seat. You will need to ensure that all child restraints are properly installed according to the manufacturer's instructions.

Plain window glass used in a car's side windows doesn't provide much protection from the sun unless a tinted ultraviolet protective film of 50+ rating is applied to the windows. If you and your baby are spending a long time in the car, then some sort of sun protection is needed, such as a shade visor on the windows, to reduce the sun exposure and to keep the heat off your little one during the drive. If your car has air-conditioning, this can help keep the air temperature cool as well.

Never leave your baby alone in the car – ever. Sometimes, when travelling in the car with your baby, you will need to stop and get out to quickly pick up something. While it might seem like a drag to get her out of her child restraint and either carry her or even put her in the pram, you must resist the temptation to leave her in the car and take 'just a minute' to run in and out of wherever you're going by yourself.

Not leaving a baby unattended in a car is especially important if it's a hot day. Once you park your car, the internal temperature rises 20 to 30 degrees hotter than the outside temperature, with the fastest rise in temperature happening in the first 5 minutes. Leaving the window open 1 centimetre at the top won't help your baby, either, as this may only reduce the temperature by 1 degree.

Your baby is too precious to leave in a car by herself, whether day or night. The hassle of the few moments of your time it takes you to undo child restraints and wrestle with prams is nothing to the lifetime of misery if something happens to her.

It's essential to take your baby with you whenever you leave your car – even for a minute. She'll be interested to see what you're doing and she can catch up on sleep later, if you're worried about her waking.

Playtime

With all that socialising during the feed, you might wonder what time is playtime. Playtime can be anytime. There is no set time to play. When you change your baby's nappy you might sing to her or count her toes – that's play. When you carry her from one end of the house to the other, you can point out the photos on the walls or look out the windows – that's socialising and learning.

Often, you're so tired it's a relief to be able to start putting your baby on the floor with a bunch of toys to look at on her own; you can usually start to give her short periods of floor play using a bouncer or chair with an exciting mobile at about 6 weeks. It's a popular belief that this is the type of play she needs after every feed. However, that's not the only playtime your baby needs. Her brain grows and develops the most through social interactions with you. You and all your loving social interactions are the most important contribution to her brain development.

Short amounts of time for floor play on her own, with you nearby, are fine and that way you get a much-needed break. As a little baby, she will probably start with holding a rattle, batting the toys on the play gym or simply having a look around; after all, everything is so new and different. As she gets older, she will have a greater attention span and be able to play with toys for longer periods.

While she has her solo play, you could have a rest, sit nearby and have lunch, morning or afternoon tea. Take advantage of those moments when she's happily occupied to rest. That way you'll have more energy for what your baby benefits from the most: tending to her when she needs you, feeding her, socialising and helping her adjust her day–night rhythms. This is what most helps with her early brain development.

She will enjoy the toys more if you join in with her after she has explored them herself. You can tell her what they are, the colour and texture. Smiling and laughing with her stimulates her brain to grow, makes her feel good and helps your relationship develop. You will also

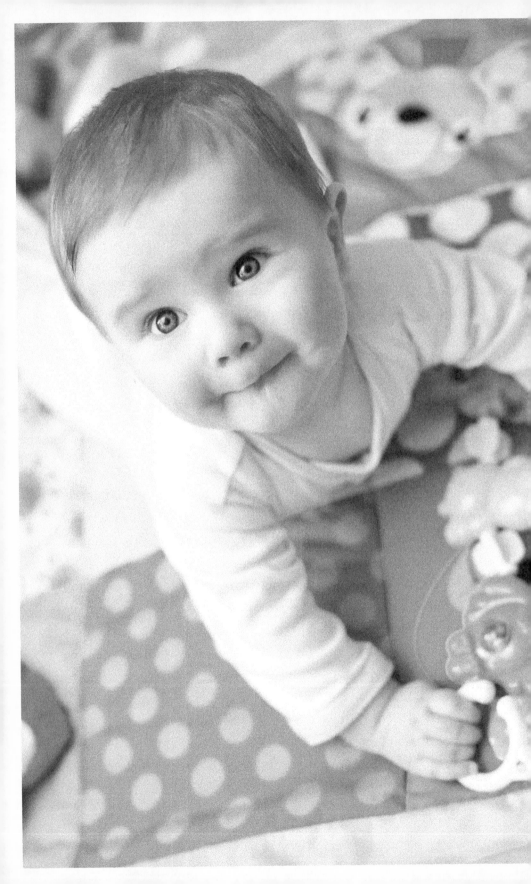

begin to recognise her non-verbal language (see Chapter 6: How your baby communicates).

The more you're with her and the longer you watch her, the quicker you will begin to recognise when she's getting overwhelmed and grumpy with playing and needs a cuddle and quiet time. By cuddling and soothing her, you lower her alertness and get her ready for a rest. You may be able to avoid some crying periods.

> By joining in social times and closely watching your baby's activity, you will become more synchronised to her rest–activity cycles and day–night cycles.

By joining in social times and closely watching your baby's activity, you will become more synchronised to her rest–activity cycles and day–night cycles and this, in turn, coordinates your baby's circadian rhythms. It gets you both ready for the next stage of sleep development: joining those sleep cycles together.

Whenever you're confused about your baby's needs or behaviour, a good way to help find an answer is to ask yourself, 'What would that be like for me?' or 'What usually happens to me in that situation?' Your baby is just a little human being who has the same feelings and needs as you. What you're learning to do is to interpret your baby's physical and emotional needs, not just for yourself but for her as well.

Caitlin's story (mother of Amelie, 4, and Maia, 1)

One of the things that's hardest prior to having your first child is the uncertainty about what is going to come. Some babies are sleepy from the very beginning, others just never seem to understand the concept of sleep and scream from the word go. Some babies love hustle and bustle and will easily drift off in the pram, others like the cool, calm quiet of their bassinet in a darkened room. Then once you think you've worked out what your baby wants, she will probably change her mind and want something else!

I had certain images of how early motherhood would be. I imagined rocking my baby to sleep in my comfy feeding chair and placing her gently in her bassinet where she would slumber for hours at a time. I imagined myself wandering up to the local shops with my baby sleeping in the pram and indulging in a well-earned cup of coffee.

None of those things came true – well, not in the first few months.

From the moment she was born, my daughter cried. She lay on my chest for the first hour with a startled expression on her face and screamed. She wailed while they weighed her, she howled while her father held her. At one point, I looked at the midwife and asked, 'Are they always like this?'

'Sometimes,' she said with a knowing smile and helped me direct my little one's mouth onto my breast. Aaah, finally some silence.

This was a pattern that continued for many weeks. I'd heard that newborns slept a lot but clearly, my daughter had not been given that memo in the womb. She hated the pram, detested the car and wasn't particularly fond of the bassinet either.

She would fall asleep in our arms, then as soon as we tried to transfer her into the cot her eyebrows would furrow and she'd let out an almighty bellow. The only place she was happy was lying on a warm body. So, as she was our first and we had nowhere else to be, we indulged her.

We spent hours lying on the couch with her slumbering in our arms. We downloaded the full series of the latest TV shows and watched them together, occasionally pausing to gaze at her as she twitched in her sleep. We bought insulated travel mugs so we could drink without spilling anything on her. When we had to leave our little nest, we took a baby carrier and let her sleep against our chest as we met up with friends or went shopping.

Admittedly, night-times could be a struggle. I remember bouncing her in my arms, willing her eyes to droop so I could attempt to lower her into her bassinet and fall exhausted into bed. The worst was when her eyes sprung open just as I'd laid her down and I'd be forced to start the whole dance again.

Nothing lasts forever, certainly not the newborn phase – although it doesn't feel like that at the time. With a lot of patience, patting and time, my daughter did learn to sleep on her own. However, I'll be forever thankful for those first few weeks when we stopped and simply enjoyed her. She was one of those babies who needed some extra cuddles to help her adjustment into the world, and we were lucky enough to be able to spare the time to give her that.

Key message

- Your baby needs plenty of natural light during the day and natural dark during the night. This helps you to synchronise your baby's sleep rhythms to the 24-hour day–night clock soon after birth.
- Daytime is social time for you and your baby. Go for walks and make sure you and your baby enjoy plenty of time socialising during nappy changes, walking from room to room and especially during feeding times. This is how your baby's brain grows and develops.
- Night-time should be dim and quiet. When you make sure that your baby has a clear and consistent bedtime, with lights out and minimal social time, she will not become overstimulated and wakeful during the night.
- Establish a routine – but be flexible! Routines for babies need to be familiar, predictable and responsive to their needs and, most importantly, flexible. Your baby will want to feed when she's hungry and needs to go to sleep when she's tired, but not by rigidly following the clock. Having a predictable bedtime routine is very important to help your baby adjust her biological rhythms to the day and night.

CHAPTER 2

Sleeping longer through the night

Did you know that in the first three years of their baby's life about 20 to 30 per cent of parents see at least one health professional for help with their child's sleep? That's a lot of tired and confused parents and babies! Know that you're not alone – other parents are struggling with exactly the same sleep worries.

There's also so much conflicting advice available. How do you know what's the right thing to do? How do you know what you're reading now is the right thing to do?

Well, that's a good question. A good way to start answering it is by helping you understand how your baby's sleep develops so you can make up your own mind about the next step you take in managing her sleep.

Having sleep difficulties with your baby is like any relationship difficulty. Both of you have to figure out what's not working and, more importantly, what is. Sometimes you both get so tired you forget how much you like to talk and cuddle with each other. That's important because talking and cuddling will help your baby sleep. Stress does not help sleep – you know that.

The problem with your relationship with your baby is she can't tell you her difficulties, so you have to do it for her. One of the best ways to understand what's going on is to wonder what it's like to be her and try to see her struggle from her point of view. This can give you some answers. Understanding her developing sleep patterns will also give you clues.

In the previous chapter, we looked at the development of your baby's first sleep rhythms. In this chapter, we focus on her second sleep rhythm, where your baby begins to sleep longer through the night.

This type of rhythm takes longer to develop, usually six to 12 months. Knowing how this second sleep rhythm develops will hopefully answer a lot of your questions about why your baby wakes so frequently. Once you understand the development of this second rhythm, you will have more ideas about how to help her.

Sleep–awake balance

Sometimes, people think that their baby needs to go to sleep when she's not ready or by a set schedule and then they wonder why she doesn't go to sleep. Your baby is just like you: she goes to sleep when she needs sleep. She definitely needs to sleep more frequently than you, but she still only needs to sleep after she's been awake for a certain period of time, depending on her age. Her brain and body will tell her when it's time to sleep.

The development of sleep is complex and is controlled by the brain and the body. Now that you've begun to figure out how circadian rhythms work, the next part of the sleep puzzle to unlock is that sleep and wakefulness also need to maintain a balance in your baby's brain. This means that her need to sleep increases the longer she's awake – this is called 'sleep pressure'.

Here's how it works. Sleep pressure builds during the time your baby is awake. Usually, she'll have a feed and some social time with you and then, after a while, she will get drowsy and feel sleepy. Drowsiness is essential before sleep and so it accompanies other tired signs. (There is more information about your baby's non-verbal cues and tired signs in Chapter 6: How your baby communicates.) Then she will fall asleep unless something, or someone, prevents her.

So, along with her circadian rhythms, your baby maintains a sleep–awake balance. This is important for you to know when it comes to recognising when she needs to go to sleep.

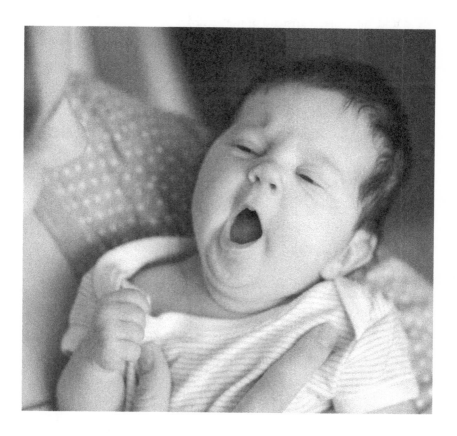

Sleep cycles explained

Apart from the day–night circadian sleep cycle, your baby has another type of sleep cycle to develop. The second sleep cycle occurs during your baby's periods of sleep.

Both the sleep and awake states have their own particular physical and behavioural patterns. Your baby's sleep cycles are divided up into two distinct 'sleep states'. You're probably familiar with the terms rapid eye movement (REM) or dream sleep, and non-rapid eye movement (non-REM) or deep sleep. These are what the adult sleep states are called. Your baby's sleep states are called 'active sleep' (dreaming) instead of REM and 'quiet sleep' instead of non-REM.

Your baby already had periods of active sleep and quiet sleep in the months before birth. You may have been aware of those times when your baby was asleep in your womb. In fact, by paying close attention to when she's asleep and awake during the last month of pregnancy, you can actually predict what her daily sleep patterns are going to be after birth.

If she's awake and busy between 2 am and 4 am, then she's likely to be wakeful around that time after she's born. The good thing about that is she's giving you a heads up while you're pregnant; that way you can be prepared and arrange your day so you can get some rest after her arrival.

Once she's born, her sleep continues to develop internally in response to her own brain and body. What's more important, her sleep is also impacted on by what's happening in her environment and how you help her to sleep. You're a team when it comes to helping your baby gradually develop her ability to sleep longer and soothe herself to sleep.

Your baby is not unconscious when she's asleep. During those early weeks when she's mostly asleep, her brain is highly active and dreaming during sleep. She needs to dream because as she isn't awake much and unable to socialise, this helps her brain to grow. But this doesn't mean you should keep her awake and socialise with her – she needs all that sleep. She will socialise at exactly the right time and when she needs to.

As she becomes more wakeful and socialises and plays with you, her social brain will get more stimulation from you and she won't have to dream as much. This means her brain is growing.

By the way, did you know that humans have a social brain? Our brain is wired up to want to be with people. The most important things you can do for your baby's brain development are to talk to her, smile, laugh, play and learn her non-verbal language so you can understand how she communicates with you (see Chapter 6: How your baby communicates).

During these early weeks, your baby has much more dream or active sleep than you do. She is different from you though, because your baby begins her sleep in active or dream sleep and then spends equal times in quiet and active sleep. These episodes of quiet and active sleep alternate for 50 to 60 minutes. This is what is generally known as a sleep cycle.

When she's younger than 3 months, your baby's active sleep is different to yours. Think about when you dream (your REM/active sleep). You don't move about much, unless you have a nightmare and wake up startled. You may wake after you dream, but you usually go back to sleep.

If you watch your baby sleep, you'll see during quiet sleep that she won't move much at all and might be difficult to rouse. During active sleep, she'll move her arms and legs, suck and smile. This can be confusing for you because you may think she's awake. Even more confusing, at the end of active sleep, you'll see that your baby usually stirs as she moves into a transitional state and seems as if she might be awake. This is when she might cry and call out. Sometimes she will manage to go back to sleep, other times she will need your help.

The most important things you can do for your baby's brain development are to talk to her, smile, laugh, play with her and learn her non-verbal language.

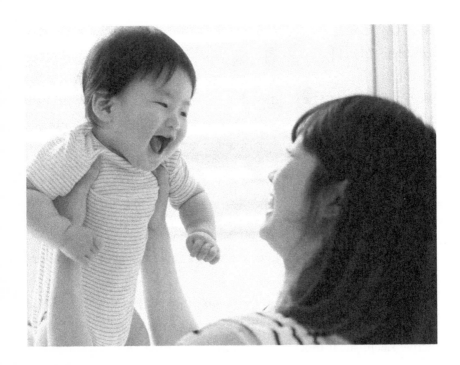

Until she's 3 months of age, her sleep cycles are still very immature, so she may not be able to self-soothe and sleep for long periods without your help. By 3 months, your baby will spend less time in active sleep during the daytime because she is awake and much more sociable. Her brain is getting stimulation from the outside world, so she doesn't need to dream so much. She spends more time in quiet sleep during the day and night, and she begins sleep in quiet sleep.

At this age, she moves her arms and legs less in active sleep, so that's less confusing for you. The more time your baby spends awake, active and sociable, the less active sleep she'll have during the day.

From 3 months, her active and quiet sleep continues to mature. Sleep cycles remain at 50 to 60 minutes in length. Her sleep changes at night as well, with quiet sleep dominating the sleep cycles at the beginning of the night and active sleep dominating the cycles in the early hours of the morning.

It's good to understand how sleep cycles work because active sleep is associated with waking and the ability to self-soothe as your baby grows and develops. This is where sleep difficulties often occur.

Now, you are probably very interested in understanding how to get your baby to sleep through the night. 'Hooray!' you say. 'At last! Please tell me what I need to do!'

Here's the problem: if you're expecting your baby to sleep 10 to 12 hours without waking, you should know that most babies don't actually do that. So, the first thing you need to understand is why your baby doesn't usually sleep 10 to 12 hours without waking through the night.

If you don't understand how your baby's sleep develops, then you might keep expecting something unrealistic of her and, when that doesn't happen, you'll feel angry, upset and disappointed. If that happens, you won't enjoy your baby. Your baby needs you to enjoy her and delight in her.

So far, we've been telling you about important internal developmental processes that are occurring in your baby's first three months, which you have no control over. We hope this will ease your mind a little because now you know that, just as your baby will develop in so many other ways, she will also develop in relation to her sleep.

On the flip side, there are lots of external influences on your baby's sleep in which you play an important role. We've already talked about circadian rhythms and melatonin and how you can help with those, so let's keep going and move on to her sleeping through the night.

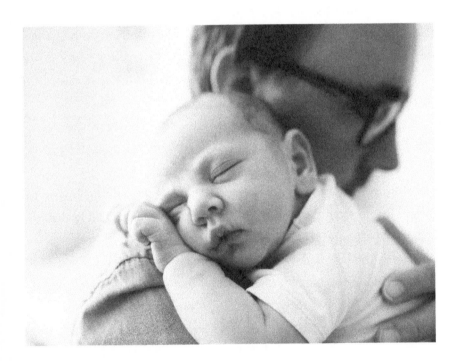

What sleeping through the night means

The importance of telling you about circadian rhythms, melatonin, the sleep–wake balance and sleep cycles first is because your baby's day–night and sleep rhythms need to be nicely established before the 'sleeping through the night' rhythms appear. These rhythms have a strong influence on the next stage of your baby's sleep development.

At first, your baby has about five to six sleep episodes evenly distributed throughout the 24-hour day. Remember, too, that for the first four to six weeks there is no day–night rhythm established yet.

At about 6 weeks, sleep begins to become more concentrated into the night-time hours and your baby is more awake during the day. By 12 weeks, your baby will have established a clear day–night pattern.

Your baby's wakeful periods will continue to increase during the day and her day sleeps will consolidate into naps. Each nap will vary in length depending on how tired your baby is and how much sleep she needs. Here's what her naps might look like:

- **6 to 9 months:** two to three daytime naps (approximately 3 to 4 hours in total throughout the day)
- **9 to 18 months:** two naps a day (approximately 2 to 3 hours in total throughout the day)
- **18 months to 3 years:** one nap in the afternoon (approximately 2 hours).

Over time, most of your baby's sleep will be at night, as the sleep–wake pattern of night sleep gradually starts to change.

'Great!' you say, 'this is when my baby will sleep through the night! I knew it!'

Yes, you're sort of right, but here's a question: what do you think 'sleeping through the night' means for a 3-month-old baby? How long would a 3-month-old baby sleep at night? Or a 6-month-old baby? What about a 12-month-old baby? Is it 12 hours, 10 hours or 8 hours?

Your answer probably depends on what you've seen on TV, read on the internet, in books or magazines, or what friends and family tell you. Whatever you've been told, the number of hours might have been overestimated.

So, how does your baby sleep through the night? And have you ever thought about what she has to be able to do to sleep through the night?

Try thinking about sleep as you would about her developing the ability to walk. You wouldn't expect your 4-month-old baby to suddenly stand up and walk. You know there are many 'steps' (LOL) she has to take before she can walk on her own. It will take months for her to walk. But it's a normal developmental task that you wait patiently to develop because you know there's a process to it.

Sleep is just the same sort of developmental process and it matures over the first six to 12 months. Sleeping through the night means different developmental milestones need to be reached, including different lengths of times asleep for different ages.

Sleeping for one 12-hour stretch through the night without waking isn't usual. It's perfectly normal for all babies from birth to 1 year of age to wake up about three times each night for 1 to 5 minutes at a time.

In the first three months, 95 per cent of babies will cry when waking and need to be resettled back to sleep, and this resettling may be separate from a feed time. By 8 months old, about 60 to 70 per cent of babies are able to self-settle after waking at night. So that leaves 30 to 40 per cent of babies who will still need some help with resettling at night.

During the second year, toddlers will usually self-settle more quickly and return to sleep with minimal help.

Your baby's day–night and sleep rhythms need to be nicely established before the 'sleeping through the night' rhythms appear.

Indicators for sleeping through the night

For your baby to sleep through the night, she must be mature enough to do these three things:

1. sustain longer periods of unbroken sleep (without waking) – this sleep pattern develops over the first three months and needs to occur before self-settling

2. be able to put herself back to sleep after she has woken from a period of sleep – this is self-settling, and your baby develops this gradually over the first year

3. be able to keep doing these for one stretch of 6 to 8 hours sometime during the night, hopefully while you are sleeping.

Sleep guidelines

Here are some average time guidelines, by age group, that your baby may sleep:

- **Newborn to 6 weeks:** six to eight regularly occurring periods of sleep, lasting 2 to 4 hours each, around the clock. Babies have short and sometimes frequent periods of wakefulness for a feed, short socialisation or resettle. The day–night pattern emerges by 4 weeks.
- **6 weeks to 3 months:** one period of sustained sleep of 4 to 5 hours during which your baby may begin to self-settle. Your baby still has one to three brief awakenings.
- **3 to 6 months:** the period of sustained night-time sleep has lengthened to 5 to 6 hours twice a night, during which your baby has the ability to self-settle. Your baby still has one to three brief awakenings in the night. However, she still may not self-settle.
- **6 to 12 months:** the period of sustained night-time sleep has lengthened to 6 hours twice a night, during which your baby has the ability to self-settle. Your baby still has one to three brief awakenings in the night. However, she still may not self-settle.
- **From 12 months:** the rate your baby sustains night-time sleep and self-settles steadily increases from 8 to 12 hours. That's the true meaning of sleeping through the night.

Awake/Feeding/Sleep guidelines

Age	Awake periods	Feeding	Sleep periods
Newborn to 6 weeks	1 to 2 hours at a time	Every 2 to 3 hours	Six to eight periods of sleep (lasting 2 to 4 hours each), occurring around the clock Your baby's day–night pattern emerges at around 4 weeks of age.
6 weeks to 3 months	1 to 2½ hours at a time	Every 2 to 4 hours	**Daytime naps:** three to four daytime naps (1 to 3 hours each) **Night-time sleep:** one longer sleep at night of 4 to 5 hours, with one to three brief awakenings during the night By 12 weeks, your baby will have an established day–night pattern.
3 to 6 months	2 to 3 hours at a time	Every 3 to 4 hours	**Daytime naps:** two or three daytime naps (3 to 4 hours in total) **Night-time sleep:** one longer sleep at night of 5 to 6 hours, with one to three brief awakenings during the night
6 to 12 months	2 to 4 hours at a time	Every 4 hours	**Daytime naps:** two daytime naps (2 to 3 hours in total) **Night-time sleep:** two longer sleeps at night of about 6 hours each, with one to three brief awakenings during the night
12 to 24 months	3 to 4 hours at a time	Normal family meal times, plus snacks	**Naps:** two daytime naps (2 to 3 hours in total), with naps steadily decreasing to one 2-hour nap in the afternoon during her second year **Night-time sleep:** the rate your baby sustains night-time sleep and her ability to self-settle during night wakings will help her steadily increase her length of sleep from 8 to 12 hours.

Remember, these are average guidelines only. Each baby is an individual and may sleep or stay awake for shorter or longer periods. It's important to watch your baby and learn her particular sleep and awake needs. If she is unwell or there's a disruption to her routine this will affect her sleep.

You can see there's a wide range of sleep needs for your newborn to toddler. For your child, these recommended hours of sleep and feeding are distributed across the day and are guidelines only. It's important to always be flexible. She hasn't read this book about how many hours she should be sleeping or when she should be eating. Just like you, your little one has her own developing individual sleep requirements. The secret is that you're helping her develop and manage her own sleep needs.

The most important thing to remember is you cannot control your baby's sleep. You can't teach or train her to sleep to a special, one-size-fits-all 'sleep prescription' you might have read in a book or found online, especially when she's less than 3 months old.

Some of these prescriptive ideas about sleep came from baby care 'experts' in the 1920s and 1930s – that's nearly a century ago! These ideas emerged again in the 1960s and are sadly still circulating now. (If you're interested, you can read about John B. Watson, who was one of these early child-rearing gurus, and his ideas on the internet.)

Research has come a long way since then and recommending babies should be made to be independent from birth and leaving them to manage on their own without help isn't a good idea.

Why your baby wakes up at night

So, why do some parents have to get up for their babies, while other parents don't seem to get up or they say they don't get up? Well, there's a reason.

After 3 months of age, most babies begin to sustain longer periods of sleep and will settle themselves back to sleep after waking. What differs between each baby is that some of them, maybe yours, will wake up at least once through the night and call out to you when she's in that transitional stage between sleeping and waking. She might be trying to self-settle but she still calls anyway. If that's your baby, she's called a 'signaller', which simply means she likes to call out to you and tell you: 'Don't forget I'm here and maybe I need some help here – not sure.'

The babies who have a reputation for sleeping through the 12 hours still wake up during their long sleep but they don't call out in the transitional stage. They are in their bed doing their own thing – they've pretty much got it sorted on most nights.

These babies are mostly able to put themselves back to sleep without any help from their parent. So, even though these babies are waking one to three times a night, they don't always call when they need to resettle. Their parents don't hear them and they will tell you, 'My baby sleeps through the night without waking.' You might feel bad and a failure.

But their baby won't sleep through every night; there will be nights when their baby is sick or she'll forget how to settle and need some help. That's normal, because most babies will continue to wake and need help on some nights of the week.

Why do some babies keep calling out when they wake up at night, while others don't? It's believed the way you put your baby to sleep and how you respond when she calls out to you at night have an effect on how she self-settles, both when you put her to sleep and when she wakes during that transitional stage during sleep cycles. The more you repeat a routine with her, the more the routine will become a positive feedback loop or a vicious circle. So, for example, if you respond very quickly every time she calls, she won't have an opportunity to self-settle.

Also, other difficulties, such as family stress, postnatal depression, anxiety, colic, gastro-esophageal reflux, medical problems and feeding difficulties, are all reasons why babies wake and call out for comfort rather than self-settle.

Night waking is normal because all babies wake at night.

And here's another thing. If you are thinking that sleeping through the night is an achievement for your baby rather than a normal developmental process, then that can change the way you feel about yourself and your baby, especially if your expectations aren't met.

Once something becomes an achievement to earn, if it's not accomplished within the timeframe you think it should be achieved in, it can become a problem and be seen as a failure for either yourself or your baby.

Sometimes it's tempting to be competitive about your baby's developmental milestones, especially about sleep. When you're participating in chats online or reading blogs or attending mothers' groups, someone's baby always wins the 'sleeping through the night competition' earlier than everyone else's.

'Achievement and competition thinking' will put a lot of pressure on your baby – especially when she can't do much about it before 3 to 6 months of age, while her sleep rhythms are maturing. This type of thinking can also lead to you wondering if there's something wrong with your baby or if you're a failure as a parent. That's not right for either of you. Parenting is hard enough without that.

Know this: night waking is normal because all babies wake at night – so night waking isn't the problem. The real difficulty is when your baby has a normal transitional wake time at night and she calls out to you. And, like all good parents, you respond to her when she calls out. She calls out, you go do something and she likes it.

So far, you still don't know what to do about the times your baby wakes during those transitional stages between sleep cycles and she calls to you. When you don't know what to do about your baby waking at night, it probably seems as if both you and your baby are participants in this situation. The thought that you might also have something to do with the way your baby sleeps may be causing you a mixture of reactions because traditionally, sleep difficulties have always been viewed as the baby's fault. She doesn't sleep and you get advice on how to fix your baby's sleep. Actually, it's not really either of you at fault, but you do have to work it out between you.

The biggest hurdle for you to overcome is to accept your baby doesn't have a problem at all. She loves it when you come to her at night when she calls. She won't stop doing that unless you help her.

You have quite a different problem; you probably don't like hearing her upset and crying, that's why you go quickly to her. Unfortunately, you don't like waking up frequently during the night, but you may have got into a night-time settling routine with her that's hard to change. So, it seems that you are the one experiencing a problem with the way your baby sleeps at night. But, in fact, you are both experiencing a problem.

If you're going to solve your sleep problems, you will need to solve them together – you may both need to stop doing a specific behaviour, and that can be hard. You're going to have to take the lead and figure out what each of you is doing that may be contributing to your lack of sleep.

There's a wide variety of difficulties that can cause sleep problems. A common one is continuing to use methods that you used for your newborn baby, such as nursing or feeding to sleep. This is a lovely, comfortable routine for both of you, but it can delay maturing sleep rhythms, such as the ability to self-settle to sleep at the beginning of the night, and then her ability to self-settle during the night when she has a normal night-waking episode.

When a difficulty such as this occurs, you need to understand what stage of sleep development your baby has reached so you can take the proper action to help you and her settle into a new bedtime and night-time routine (see chapters 7 to 10).

Usually, changing your sleep and settling routine to another one takes time and quite a bit of effort for you both, but especially for your baby. Remember, she's happy with the current arrangement and loves being with you, so she will protest while you both get used to a new routine. Gradually, with gentle and consistent encouragement, your baby will adjust. Just keep in mind that this new sleep and settling routine needs to be consistent with her developmental sleep age.

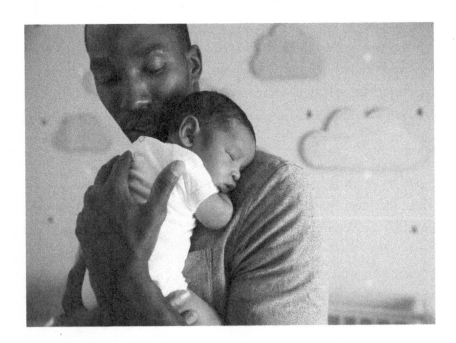

Stephanie's story (mother of Eva, 1)

I am someone who needs lots of sleep, so I was pretty concerned about how I would go waking up to my baby multiple times a night. Initially, it was tough waking up and feeding when Eva cried, but it's amazing how quickly you get used to broken sleep. In the first few months, she woke two or three times a night and I actually grew to enjoy that time. I would sit in my feeding chair with her wrapped up in my arms and I'd usually take the chance to read some emails or do a bit of online shopping! It was like we were the only people in the world and it felt warm and comforting.

However, after four or five months the novelty was wearing off. Some of my friends in my mothers' group had started talking about how their babies were sleeping through the night. They'd put them down at 7 pm and they wouldn't hear a peep out of them until 7 am.

'You hear that?' I'd say to Eva. 'Sam is sleeping all night long and you are still waking up at least twice. How about you get some tips!'

I felt like a bit of a failure that she wasn't sleeping through the night. Some of my other friends decided to sleep train and all swore by it. They said there were a few difficult nights but the results were worth it – their babies had slept 12 hours every night since. It was something I really wrestled with. I really wanted sleep but I just didn't feel ready to go through a sleep training method with Eva. I was hoping that she'd get there when she was ready and that it would be soon!

I wondered if she was hungry, so I decided to start solids. She loved food and took to it with gusto, eating everything I gave her. However, after a few months she was still waking at least twice for a feed. Sometimes she woke up at 10 pm or 11 pm, then again at around 4 am. Other times, she slept through until 1 am or 2 am, then woke again at 5 am. Luckily, the feed was fast – just 10 or 15 minutes, then she'd be straight back to sleep, but I was still tired. Weren't babies meant to be sleeping through the night by 7 months?

I remember going to the Early Childhood Centre and talking to a nurse. She listened to all my concerns, we went through our evening routine and spoke about the times when Eva woke up. She said I was doing everything right, but often breastfed babies weren't ready to give up those night feeds just yet.

At about 9 months, Eva started waking later and later for her first feed. Sometimes it was 2 am, then it was 3 am. The second feed became the morning feed at 6 am or 7 am. Then all of a sudden, one night she didn't wake at all! The next night she did the same and I realised we'd done it – our baby was sleeping through the night!

Now she's 1 and she sleeps through the night every night. There's a lot of pressure to have a 'good' baby that sleeps through the night at an early age, but I actually think it's okay to just have a 'normal' baby who sleeps through when she is ready.

Key message

- Sleep difficulties with your baby are like every relationship difficulty – you just need to figure out what the problem is.
- Sleep is a developmental process that matures over the first six to 12 months.
- All babies wake at night, the difference is whether your baby calls out to you.

CHAPTER 3

The two sides of your sleep problems

There are two sides to sleeping problems – yours and your baby's. You might be saying, 'Yes, and my side is that I'm sleep deprived because my baby won't let me sleep!' There's no denying that's true, but the problem is a bit more complicated than that.

Because you're so tired and eager for answers, it seems much easier to go for a quick fix, right? Then, when that doesn't work, you blame yourself or your baby. Something must be wrong with one of you. Well, in truth, it's not actually anyone's fault, and there are reasons for that.

Traditionally, all sleep problems have been blamed solely on the baby, so any sleep approach has usually been to 'fix' a baby's sleep. You might have been given many ideas on how to 'fix' her sleep but those solutions might not have worked for you. Strategies to 'fix' sleep problems are usually focused on your baby's biological sleep processes but often overlook that you and your baby have many emotions that also affect sleep.

So, seeing as there are two sides to why any sleep difficulties might occur and persist, it's best to first consider some of the difficulties you might be experiencing that could be playing a part in the challenges around sleep.

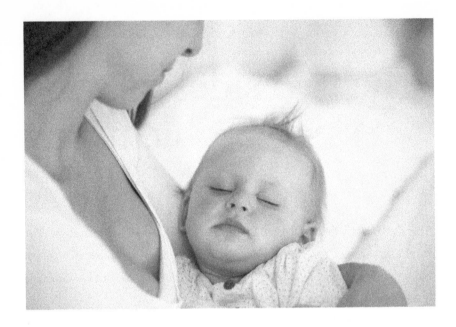

There are a number of reasons why some sleep approaches don't produce the results parents were hoping to see in certain circumstances. The approach may not have taken into account such important things as:

- your baby's different stages of sleep development
- your baby's very close and dependent relationship with you
- the importance of you and your baby working together on her daily rhythms of sleeping, feeding and socialising
- how much family support you have
- what's going on in your home environment
- your and your baby's health.

Before going any further in this chapter, it's probably a good idea to refresh your memory about the ages your baby begins to self-settle and sleep for longer periods through the night. That way you can make a quick reference to self-settling and sleep times if you need to while you read this chapter.

Sleep guidelines

Here are some average time guidelines, by age group, that your baby may sleep:

- **Newborn to 6 weeks:** six to eight regularly occurring periods of sleep, lasting 2 to 4 hours each, around the clock. Babies have short and sometimes frequent periods of wakefulness for a feed, short socialisation or resettle. The day–night pattern emerges by 4 weeks.
- **6 weeks to 3 months:** one period of sustained sleep of 4 to 5 hours during which your baby may begin to self-settle. Your baby still has one to three brief awakenings.
- **3 to 6 months:** the period of sustained night-time sleep has lengthened to 5 to 6 hours twice a night, during which your baby has the ability to self-settle. Your baby still has one to three brief awakenings in the night. However, she still may not self-settle.
- **6 to 12 months:** the period of sustained night-time sleep has lengthened to 6 hours twice a night, during which your baby has the ability to self-settle. Your baby still has one to three brief awakenings in the night. However, she still may not self-settle.
- **From 12 months:** the rate your baby sustains night-time sleep and self-settles steadily increases from 8 to 12 hours. That's the true meaning of sleeping through the night.

Sleeping for one 12-hour stretch through the night without waking isn't usual. It's perfectly normal for all babies from birth to 1 year of age to wake up about three times each night for 1 to 5 minutes at a time.

Ideas are powerful

You have probably read or been told by friends and family all sorts of information about how babies should sleep. All this information can be confusing. Who's right, and who's wrong?

Some people say babies should be taught to sleep through the night from birth, others tell you to let your baby cry to sleep, and there are books that tell you not to let your baby cry. Some information tells you babies should sleep 12 hours a night at 6 months of age, while others insist that babies should start to sleep through the night at 3 months. Whether you're aware of it or not, these ideas can give you unrealistic expectations of your baby, which can cause you great disappointment when they don't happen.

When you're disappointed, it's natural to feel that your baby isn't normal or you are doing something wrong. These ideas can make you doubt your competence as a parent.

And the confusion all the different opinions cause can lower your confidence in making decisions about caring for your baby, which in turn can lead to other negative feelings, such as resentment or anger at your baby's demands. Then like a chain reaction, this causes you more guilt and distress because you doubt your ability to care for your baby as well as other parents do. You might also feel that your baby isn't as 'good' or 'well behaved' as other babies, and then you might feel guilt for feeling angry or negative towards your baby. Sometimes, you can get caught in a vicious circle of feelings and behaviour, and it feels awful!

This cycle of negative feelings is a common problem for parents and can happen because of the enormous amount of misleading and sometimes incorrect information written about babies and their sleep. These mixed ideas can come from mainstream media, books, websites and well-meaning friends and family. Some of the mainstream material is not well researched, is personal opinion or just simply outdated information.

The problem is that many of these ideas can be unrealistic for both you and your baby and very difficult to achieve if your baby isn't mature enough. Most importantly, though, these ideas can affect your relationship with each other. Anything that affects your relationship with your baby not only makes sleep difficulties worse, but feeding and socialising and play can be negatively affected as well.

You and your baby

If the information you're reading or hearing doesn't tell you about your baby's sleep development and give you strategies that match your baby's developmental stage, then it's probably not helpful. Information that focuses solely on 'fixing' your baby isn't fair to your baby or you. You need to understand your baby's personality, age and development so you won't be disappointed and become stressed out if your baby is not achieving what the advice you're reading says she's supposed to be doing.

Any information you read should also consider you and your baby's situation. This includes how you are feeling, what support you have available, how you are settling your baby and what you have found helpful for you both. This is very important because you and your baby are a team.

There isn't a 'one size fits all' approach to sleep problems. You and your baby are different from other parents and their babies, so you will need to be flexible in your approach. Once again, think about the way you sleep. Perhaps you could ask your partner or a friend how they sleep and compare each other's sleep patterns and habits. Ask your parent if he or she remembers how you slept as a baby. Did you wake frequently through the night like your baby or were you able to self-settle? Maybe you were an early riser. If you have siblings, you could ask your parent what sort of 'sleepers' they were. Sometimes other family members have similar stories of 'night-wakers'. Everyone sleeps differently; your baby does too. What you have to do is help her develop her own healthy, individual sleep habits.

Getting up at night when you hear your baby

Like many parents, you may find it difficult not to jump up to every sound and squeak that comes from your baby or if she calls out while preparing to go back into another sleep cycle. Some parents have said this is because they:

- are worried they are being insensitive
- are worried they are being neglectful
- would feel guilty
- have trouble setting limits.

They also have the idea their baby is:

- frightened
- anxious
- lonely.

Sometimes, you're not aware that you have these types of ideas or worries. Take some time to think about it. This might help you to understand why you feel a certain way when you hear your baby making sounds. Some parents find themselves running to their baby to stop her becoming distressed, even when there is no sign that is going to happen.

It's important to consider your responses, because the way you're thinking and feeling about why your baby is waking at night can interfere with finding ways to solve your sleep difficulties. And it may have also affected any previous methods you've tried.

If you're now discovering that you are thinking a particular way, consider how those thoughts might be preventing you from helping your baby to go to sleep and stay asleep. This is the first thing to do before beginning to think about ways to help your baby to self-settle by her developmental sleep age.

The way you're thinking and feeling about why your baby is waking at night can interfere with finding ways to solve your sleep difficulties.

A common reason for going to your baby when you hear her at night is that you are afraid your baby is frightened, anxious or lonely and needs your immediate help. Does that sound like you?

It's understandable that you would feel guilty, insensitive and neglectful if you didn't go and help her immediately when you believe your baby is frightened, anxious or lonely. But the truth is when your baby wakes normally at night, and she's not crying but simply making little noises or even a small 'hey' as she tries to go back to sleep, then she's usually not frightened, anxious or lonely. She is probably missing you because she loves you, but she still needs you to give her a little opportunity to try and self-settle back to sleep. If you're anxious and distressed when you go to her quickly, when she wakes she will pick up on your anxiety and is more likely to be anxious. She won't know what she's anxious about; her instinct will just alert her to maintain contact with you.

The reason she is waking up is because it's developmentally normal for her wake one to three times a night, make some sounds and then try to resettle back to sleep. Unfortunately, when you have the idea that she might be frightened, anxious or lonely, you're more likely to go to your baby as soon as you hear her wake. You become involved in very frequent, active soothing during the night, which may overstimulate her rather than soothe her. This means she doesn't get a chance to try to self-settle and will rely on you to go back to sleep.

Examples of active soothing

Active soothing, which may interfere with your baby's chances
of learning to self-settle, includes such things as:

- picking your baby up as soon as she wakes
- rocking her in your arms
- feeding back to sleep
- co-sleeping
- overexposure to blue light during the night
- too much handling or overstimulation.

Set limits on yourself

When your baby wakes and calls, wait to see if she resettles. Listen to her
carefully; while she's making small grunts, snorts, little sounds and calls
just leave her. When you respond to your baby straight away with active
settling strategies, without giving her an opportunity to self-settle, you
tend to wake her up even more. Once she starts to fuss a little bit that's
when you respond and provide settling strategies (see chapters 7 to 10).

However, if she becomes very fussy and distressed she will be
much harder to settle as well. It's essential to respond to her quickly
so you can soothe and calm her. If she becomes very distressed, have
a look at the strategies for soothing a crying baby in Chapter 5: Why
your baby cries.

In the meantime, when you try and wait while your baby is making
little sounds to see if she's going to settle by herself, you're setting a limit
on yourself. That means you're resisting your urge to get up and go to
her even though you desperately want to.

To help you wait while she tries to settle, you could say to yourself,
'She's okay, she's just trying to go back to sleep. I'm the one who's
feeling anxious.'

If you find waiting really hard, this could mean you are having some difficulty setting limits on yourself because you are so worried she's frightened, anxious or lonely. That's why you respond so quickly to her calls. This is common for some parents. What your baby needs you to do is to try to hold yourself back from going to her until you're sure she's not going to settle herself and has started to really fuss for you.

When you've decided she really needs your help, go to her, but try not to pick her up. Keep her in her bed and gently and sensitively see what she needs. It may be as simple as your soothing calm voice, a gentle pat or rub on her tummy, or a stroke on her head, while you say 'shhh, shhh'. This behaviour is responsive to her needs. What she needs is to be simply calmed back to sleep without too much stimulation.

This is quite a balancing act, trying to wait to go to her until exactly the right moment between fussing and all-out crying! But if you really listen carefully and begin to learn about your baby and the types of messages she sends to you when she needs your help at night, eventually, you'll help her manage to self-settle.

Depending on her age, refer to chapters 7 to 10 for ways to settle your child to sleep, from birth through to preschooler years.

Anxiety

Feeling constantly anxious can cause you to get up too quickly to tend to your baby when she calls out at night. Everyone feels anxious sometimes and that's totally normal, but constant anxiety isn't good for you or your baby. There are a number of reasons why you might be feeling constantly anxious. You might:

- be feeling generally anxious and worried about your baby
- be feeling anxious about separating from your baby
- be anticipating the times your baby will wake up and cry so you can't sleep properly
- be constantly checking on your baby because you aren't sleeping well, even when she does sleep
- have postnatal depression and/or anxiety.

Anxiety is a very uncomfortable experience for you and your baby. It can happen when you:

- lose a lot of sleep
- are not feeling good about yourself
- have tried lots of sleep approaches and nothing works
- feel like a failure as a parent
- are worried about your baby
- have postnatal depression and/or anxiety.

The problem with a constant state of anxiety is that it doesn't just affect you. When you care for your baby in an anxious state, she will feel your anxiety and may become anxious as well. She won't know why you're anxious, but the anxiety translates to her as messages that something is wrong, unsafe or uncomfortable.

When your baby senses something is wrong or unsafe, her instinct tells her to stay close to you. She will cling to you. She will want you to hold her and keep her safe. This comes from our human evolution, and it's important to understand this from your baby's point of view.

Babies and children don't know what's dangerous; they rely on their parents to show them. Your baby is highly attuned to your emotional state and ready to run away from danger with you. She can't walk yet, so she has to cling on in case you leave. If she's not clinging on, she has to cry and call for you.

As long as she senses from you that something might be wrong or unsafe, she won't want you to put her down and she will cry and fuss for you. She needs to be with you for safety and comfort. She's not being naughty – her instincts are telling her to keep close and safe with you, her favourite person in the whole world.

Unfortunately, the anxiety you feel translates messages that don't help your efforts to aid her settle to sleep. She doesn't want you to leave her alone and she may well be anxious or frightened.

What you can do

One of the most helpful ways of solving sleep problems is becoming aware of the reasons why you are getting up to your baby at night. When you understand how you're thinking about a problem and the reasons why you're doing certain things, you have the key to finding a new approach or modifying some of the approaches you've already tried.

Try paying more attention to the types of ideas you might be having about why you get up to your baby at night. Sometimes just thinking them through quietly on your own can be enough to help you make sense of them. If that's not enough, you could talk with your family or a close, safe friend who's able to help you think about your ideas. You might also discover you're not alone in your thinking.

If you are having problems with your baby's sleep, then one of the best things you can do is to find someone to support you. You need someone who is able to reassure you that your baby is not frightened or anxious and that you're not being neglectful or insensitive while you give her the space to settle by herself in her crib. This could be your partner, mother, sister, aunt, friend or a parenting centre. If you need help with sleep and settling strategies, look at chapters 7 to 10, which cover birth to preschool.

If you've realised that you are constantly anxious or frightened about leaving your baby to sleep or to try to settle by herself, then this can be a difficult and unhappy situation for both of you. It's very important to talk to someone close to you to get support and reassurance. If you are constantly feeling anxious and recognise that your baby doesn't like to be put down, it's probably best to talk with a health professional to ensure your anxiety is well managed and to see if you require counselling and/ or medication.

Avoiding high levels of continuous anxiety is important for both you and your baby. Anxiety can be sorted out with help and support. And this will help you and your baby to enjoy each other so much more.

Quick ways to soothe yourself

There are some really quick and easy ways to help soothe yourself if you are feeling anxious.

Manage your breathing. Have you ever thought about how you are breathing when you're anxious? Do you hold your breath and you're not aware you're doing that?

Take time to notice how you're breathing. Are you taking little, shallow breaths from the top of your chest? Put your hands there and feel it.

That's not nearly enough oxygen for you and your brain. Holding your breath and taking shallow breaths doesn't help you feel good or think clearly.

When you're feeling anxious, deep breathing can help you to feel calmer. It can clear your head, give you more oxygen and help you focus your thoughts.

Calm breathing technique

1. Put your hands just below both sides of your rib cage and close your eyes.
2. Focus on taking in a slow breath through your nose as you count to three.
3. Gently breathe in so you can feel your breath lift your rib cage under your hands and your stomach pull inwards. Don't breathe in too deeply or hold your breath – you don't want to get dizzy.
4. Then breathe out slowly through your mouth while you count to three.
5. Keep your eyes closed and just focus on your breathing.

Repeat this technique two more times and then stop and relax. Deep breathing is a great way calm down. You can do deep breathing anytime you feel anxious. And it's especially good to do before you go to your baby if you are in an anxious state already.

Get moving. Stress responses in the body involve the release of chemical messages in the brain and hormones, such as cortisol – the 'fight or flight' response. Your body does this when there's danger. When you're constantly anxious, your body is having a 'fight or flight' response for absolutely no reason.

People who are anxious release 'fight or flight' response chemicals and hormones at the wrong times. As you can imagine, if you are feeling the need to 'fight or flight' then trying to rest, sleep and enjoy normal activities is going to be difficult.

If that's what you're experiencing, then it's best not to sit still. When you are anxious and your body is telling you to 'fight or flight' without any good reason, don't fight it. The stress chemicals are telling you to run, so it's the time to do anything vigorous that uses up the overactive stress response. You will feel better.

It could be as easy as:

- a quick walk
- a round of stretching
- climbing up and down some stairs a few times
- touching your toes or doing some sit-ups.

All you need to do is any quick and easy exercise that uses up that anxious energy and makes you feel better.

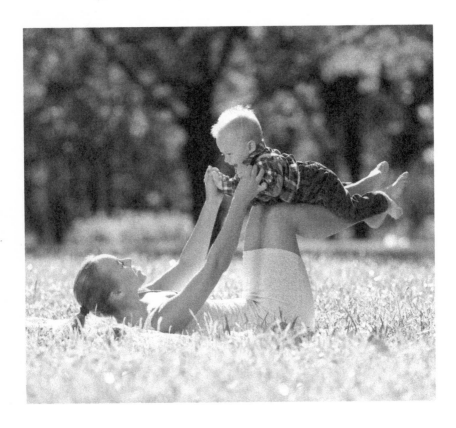

Why your baby wakes at night

Now let's take a look at what's happening for your baby and her side of your sleep problems. Here are some common but old-fashioned reasons people might have told you why your baby is waking – and note that none of them is true:

- She's being naughty.
- She's doing it to annoy you.
- She's doing it to get attention – in a naughty way.
- She's being stubborn.

As you know by now, sleep is a normal developmental process and the reason why your baby is waking up at night or between sleep cycles isn't because she's naughty or stubborn. She is definitely not doing it to annoy you or get your attention.

First of all, your baby doesn't have the ability to make plans to annoy you. Her brain is too immature to think like you do. She doesn't think in words because she doesn't have any language.

Your baby lives in a world of feelings, tastes, smells, touch and sights. That's how she gets all her information. She doesn't have a long memory either. When you leave her, she doesn't know where you've gone or when you'll come back. She simply doesn't know how to be deliberately naughty, annoy you or be stubborn.

That doesn't mean you won't feel annoyed that you have to keep getting up to her when she wakes up and calls. The main thing is, your baby has no ability whatsoever to deliberately make a plan to annoy you. Teenagers do that.

As for getting your attention – well yes, she is doing that. But is it really naughty for a young baby who can't walk, talk or help herself yet to call for you when she needs you? She's in a strange and new world. She needs lots of hugs and reassurance.

Calling and crying is the way your baby gets your attention because she doesn't have any other way to ask for your help, and she only does it when she needs to. That's what she's doing when she wakes. She doesn't know how to get back to sleep without your help.

Calling and crying is the way your baby gets your attention because she doesn't have any other way to ask for your help.

Your baby needs you to think about this from her point of view because she can't tell you her side, yet. She doesn't understand this is a problem for both of you. Remember, waking up after a sleep cycle is normal for her. Some babies may self-settle back to sleep, but you happen to have a baby who calls to you. This may be because:

- She has less mature sleep–wake patterns than other babies her age and it's going to take her a little longer to self-settle and sustain longer periods of sleep.
- You are responding a bit too quickly to her when she wakes, and then trying to settle her with active settling strategies before they are needed.

The following scenario is a common one.

Scenario: calling out to you at night

You may or may not have a bedtime routine with your baby. A common routine would be a bath, pyjamas, stories, rocking, singing and feeding her to sleep. This might be quite a long routine. Your baby may then sleep for 2 to 3 hours.

When your baby wakes up from one of her normal sleep cycles, it's dark, she's on her own and she misses all those nice bedtime routines you do. She really likes you being with her when she wakes up at night because you provide her with all the nice, comforting bedtime routines – feeding, rocking or singing her back to sleep.

This is the problem. Your baby hasn't had to develop her own ways of self-settling, so once she wakes up she has to call out for your help to get back to sleep. When you come to her, she's very glad to see you, but probably just as tired and grumpy as you. She's having broken sleep as well.

The difficulty for you is that she doesn't know how tired you are or that she's woken you up three times already. She doesn't have the capacity to consider your point of view yet. Children only learn that after they experience someone considering their point of view first. That's empathy.

So, your little baby can't empathise with you or make any decisions about the problem you both have; she just feels she needs you to go through the usual routine that helps her go to sleep, so instinctively she calls for you. You don't know how else to get her to go back to sleep either, so you go through the usual routine as well.

Both of you have developed a night-time routine, it's just that it's not helpful to do this routine again in the middle of the night.

As you can see, there's so much more to putting your baby to sleep than just wrapping her up, popping her in her crib and hoping she learns to go to sleep!

Any sleep difficulties you have are always a shared concern between you and your baby, and when you want to solve your difficulty, you are the one who always takes the lead. Sleep problems are not only struggles with your baby's biological sleep development: how you and your baby feel emotionally can affect your sleep.

Your baby's biological sleep development plays an important role in her ability to self-settle and, eventually, sleep through the night. When you understand the parameters of normal sleep development, as well as begin to learn your baby's own individual sleep needs, her sleep won't be so confusing.

The emotional difficulties can be caused by the types of ideas you get about your baby's sleep from the media and other people, your anxiety, your ability to set limits for yourself at night when you want to respond to your baby, as well as the types of settling strategies you use when your baby wakes at night.

When you understand that both you and your baby have a part to play in your sleep difficulties, it can make it easier to find a solution. If you really understand your thoughts and emotions that are often hiding beneath your sleep problems, this can make the changes easier for both you and your baby, and they are more likely to work.

Louise's story (mother of Jamie, 11 months)

Naively, I thought I had prepared myself reasonably well for having a baby. I had read a few parenting books and had lots of friends with kids. People warned me that it was hard when a baby doesn't sleep but you don't really think it will apply to you. You can't ever imagine the relentlessness of it, the day-in, day-out exhaustion and the feeling of not having a clue how to fix the problems.

My son Jamie would cry every time I put him down. Every single time. By the time he was 10 weeks old, I was at the point of wondering why on earth I had ever wanted to become a parent. I was struggling and was completely exhausted.

I was referred to the Tresillian Day Services, where the nurses showed me how to deal with his sleep issues. They taught me to settle him in my arms until he was drowsy, then place him in the cot and pat him until he went to sleep. That worked for us, and I went home feeling much happier. He was napping well during the day and started sleeping through at night. All was good!

However, about three months later everything changed. After sleeping through from 7 pm until 7 am, he started waking hourly. I had been getting pretty decent sleep for a few months and I just couldn't cope with the sudden constant wakings. I'm not proud to admit it, but I turned into a crazy person.

I started googling for information, I read all the mummy blogs and forums trying in vain to work out what might work. I tried a few things but nothing seemed to help him sleep, and I lost confidence in my ability to settle him. I went back to my doctor and she said, 'You have to go back to Tresillian.'

This time, I went to the Residential Stay for five nights. Jamie had recently started to flip himself over and sleep on his tummy, but I was paranoid about the SIDS risk, so would try to turn him onto his back and settle him that way. The first thing I learned was that if he's strong enough to roll over, he's okay to sleep on his tummy if he wants.

The support from the nurses overnight was just so incredible. They were on hand to help whenever he woke and would go through each of the stages with me. They taught me which of his cries were just whinges and which ones were real distress. Then they would help me with how to settle him, when to stop swaying and put him in his cot, and when to leave the room. In the end, I could just put him in his cot and leave the room without him crying at all. It was amazing.

I do think part of the problem was my anxiety and my lack of understanding of what was normal. I just got so tired and irrational, then I started second-guessing myself about how to settle him. I ended up being really inconsistent, following bits of advice I'd read online, then changing my mind the next day and trying something else.

I felt pressure to work out his sleep problems by myself, but that's so unrealistic. It's completely normal for babies to change their sleep habits from time to time, and I've learned not to get used to anything.

Key message

- There are two sides to the sleep problem: your baby's and yours.
- One of the most helpful ways of solving sleep problems is to become aware of the reasons why you are getting up to your baby at night.
- Everyone sleeps differently. Your baby has to learn how to self-settle before she can sleep through the night.

CHAPTER 4

Creating a conducive sleep environment

'Why a whole chapter on sleep environment?' you might be asking. Well, it's very important. Where you sleep and the conditions you like when you go to sleep are as equally important as how sleep develops.

Think about this: you have your own familiar room with a comfy bed, favourite pillows and covers. You go to your room when you want to sleep because you feel safe there. When you wake up, you expect to still be there, nice and safe in your comfortable, familiar surroundings. You need this because when you sleep, you're not alert to your surroundings, so you need to feel secure in order to relax.

Your baby is just the same as you. She needs her own safe, comfy room and bed. She also needs to be put to sleep in the same bed and room both day and night. This will help her night-time sleep.

So, sleep environment and location are very important.

Sleep location

There's lots of advice on where your baby should sleep after she's born. Some people recommend that you share a room with your baby, and other people advise that it's better to let your baby sleep in her own room. Cultural differences play a large part in choosing where you put your baby to sleep. Western cultures tend to place emphasis on encouraging independence in young children, therefore babies sleeping in their own room has become popular. Parents across other cultural groups may place less emphasis on independence, so solitary sleeping is not so important.

Co-sleeping or bed-sharing is not recommended due to the risk of Sudden Unexpected Death in Infancy (SUDI). The term SUDI includes Sudden Infant Death Syndrome (SIDS) and other fatal sleeping accidents.

Some parents do choose to co-sleep or bed-share because of their personal beliefs. Often bed-sharing happens by default – that is, you don't intend to co-sleep with your baby but you're so exhausted from frequent night waking that bed-sharing is your last resort, just to get some rest.

Whatever reason co-sleeping or bed-sharing occurs, make sure you are aware of the Red Nose SUDI guidelines (rednose.com.au/article/is-it-safe-to-sleep-with-my-baby) to ensure your baby sleeps safely.

Co-sleeping guidelines

- Sharing a sleep surface increases the risk of SIDS and fatal sleep accidents. Babies most at risk are those who are under 3 months of age, were born prematurely or were small for their gestational age.
- You shouldn't sleep with your baby on your sofa or couch, a waterbed, hammock or a beanbag. These surfaces aren't flat or stable and are completely unsafe if you fall asleep and accidentally roll on your baby.
- It's safest not to share your bed or any sleep surface with your baby and anyone who is affected by alcohol or other drugs – that includes medicines that cause drowsiness, even prescribed or over-the-counter medicines – or with someone who smokes.

Red Nose SUDI guidelines recommend you sleep your baby in your room for the first six to 12 months.

Putting your baby in a cot next to or near your bed is the safest and best sleeping arrangement for the first six to 12 months. In fact, approximately 70 per cent of parents share their room with their baby from birth. By 1 year old, about two-thirds of parents have moved their baby to their own room.

Some of the benefits your baby may gain from room-sharing with you are that you are able to monitor her wellbeing during sleep, it's easier to breastfeed or formula feed, and you can help her return to sleep more quickly after waking. You and your baby will also experience a greater sense of emotional closeness and wellbeing, and room-sharing helps with successful breastfeeding. Always return your baby to her bed after a feed; this is safest for her and will help with her settling and ability to soothe herself to sleep.

Even though Red Nose SUDI guidelines recommend you continue to sleep your baby in your room for the first six to 12 months, you might decide to move her during the second half of the year. There are all sorts of reasons you might choose to do that, among them that you might need to try to get more sleep, you want to see if your baby will sleep better in her own room, or your bedroom may be too small for a cot.

If you do choose to move your baby to her own room between 6 and 12 months, she may learn to self-settle more quickly when she wakes at night. This is because you're less likely to hear her when she rouses and calls you, so she'll have more time to try to self-settle. The downside is you may only hear her if she cries, so it's possible that if she sleeps alone she may cry more.

Negative sleep associations

Whether your baby shares your room or sleeps in her own room, it's important to consider what else affects her sleep development. Sleep problems are commonly associated with:

- lack of a consistent, relaxing and familiar bedtime routine
- irregular daily routines
- exciting activities at bedtime
- a very busy household
- having a TV in the same room your baby is sleeping in
- smartphones, tablets and computers at bedtime.

Predictable daily routines

Preparing your baby for night-time sleep isn't just about having a consistent, relaxing and soothing bedtime routine. Having familiar daily routines will provide your baby with a predictable and stress-free atmosphere during the day, which will prepare her for the night and sleep.

You know yourself how hard it can be to wind down and relax when you've had a busy, stressful day, especially if your day hasn't gone as planned and your routine has been upset. You might have been late for work and missed your lunchbreak because of some unexpected deadline. You know the type of events that completely stress you and spoil your day.

Predictable routines are not just important for your baby, they are important to you as well. One of the difficulties you may be having is that you're trying to maintain your old routine and fit your new baby around that. Unfortunately, this doesn't always work. And that can make you feel even more stressed.'

John B. Watson, an early-20th century childcare expert, said that 'babies and children should never inconvenience adults'. His old-

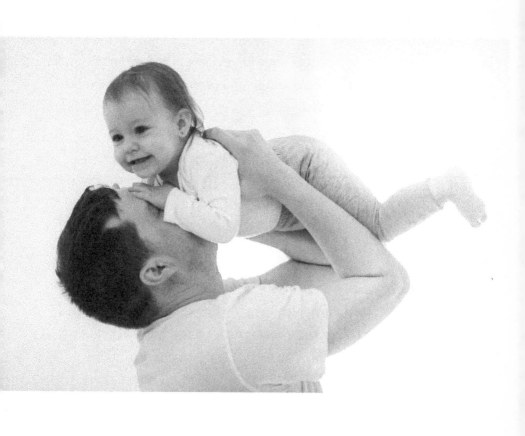

fashioned advice still influences lots of the information that's around today. Fortunately, current research understands your baby's needs much better than such old ideas.

In the meantime, your baby really can't function on an adult's routine, it's far too stressful for her. She relies on you to adjust your routine to help her establish her day–night rhythms and sleep cycles, and provide predictable and sensitive feeding and socialising times during the day.

By implementing routines you will feel more in control and that will make you feel much more confident as a parent. Better still, if it helps your baby sleep, you will sleep.

Predictable routines are not just important for your baby, they are important to you as well.

That doesn't mean you can't enjoy an active social life. You can work around your baby's developing daily rhythms and schedule enriching outings that you both enjoy. Relaxing together will help you both sleep.

So, what is a routine?

A routine doesn't mean 'by the clock'; for example, doing things at exactly 6 am, 10 am, 2 pm, 6 pm, etc. Hardly anyone lives their life like that. Your baby's routine will be organised around her feed and sleep times, and will change progressively as she matures. Basically, a routine is a series of activities done in the same order, each day.

Bedtime routines

Your baby's bedtime routine is important to help her settle. Think about your own bedtime routine. After dinner and evening chores are done, you may relax after a long busy day and watch some TV or read until you feel drowsy. You always feel drowsy before you go to sleep. You also give non-verbal cues, such as yawning, moving around restlessly, rubbing your face or sighing. You might have a warm shower, clean your teeth, change into your pyjamas, read a little and go to bed. That's a fairly common routine.

Your baby's night-time routine can be as simple as three or four steps carried out in the same order.

Consistent and familiar routines get your mind and body relaxed and ready for sleep. If you think about it, it's harder to go to sleep when your routine is disrupted, such as when you go on holiday or stay at a friend's house, or you go out to a party and come home really hyped up. It's also harder to sleep if you're anxious or worried, or you've had an argument with someone just before you go to bed.

Your baby is just the same. She, too, needs a consistent, relaxing and familiar night-time sleep routine. She needs this routine even more than you because she is developing her sleep rhythms and habits.

Her night-time routine can be as simple as three or four steps carried out in the same order over a short period of time. Depending on the age of your baby or child, the bedtime routine can take up to 30 minutes. The routine helps your baby to wind down and relax so she can fall asleep more quickly and stay asleep longer.

The type of routine is also dependent on age. You might like to include a massage in your baby's routine for the first 12 months. But your older toddler or preschooler may not enjoy a massage and would prefer stories, cuddling, singing or other quiet, soothing activities. Avoid irritability and anger at bedtime, as this causes stress and your baby, toddler or preschooler is unlikely to settle.

Sample bedtime routine

A quiet, soothing bedtime routine builds the foundation for a good sleep, helping your baby to fall asleep faster and stay asleep longer. There is no set time for bedtime – this is up to you and what's right for you culturally and personally.

1. Give your baby a bath – this is always soothing and relaxing and improves sleep. Typically, her bath should be before her first night-time sleep.
2. Try giving her a gentle massage with an oil (for babies under 12 months and only if she enjoys it – some babies don't like such intense touching).
3. Put her in her pyjamas.
4. Using a soft, low and quiet voice, read stories or rhymes, sing songs and/or lullabies to her.
5. Give her plenty of calm cuddles.
6. Place your baby on her back in her own bed.
7. Turn out the lights and leave the room.

Morning routines

Consistency in establishing sensitive and responsive routines throughout the day and night is known to help babies and children sleep through the night.

This routine doesn't run to a time on the clock. It will depend on when your baby wakes from a sleep and ends when she shows you she's tired and ready for bed. The routine is a series of activities done in the same order in a predictable, sensitive and responsive way. Putting in place a routine like this will help you and your baby have more stress-free days and nights.

Having a baby does change your old routines significantly and it can be a shock to find that someone so little can change your life so completely. This is especially true if you were led to believe that your baby would just fit in with your old lifestyle.

Thank goodness your baby is so delightful and melts your heart with each smile, or reaches out to you for a hug or laughs maniacally at you when you hide your head under her blankie. And what about those funny, gummy kisses on your chin! She always has an ace up her sleeve to help you both get over those glitches.

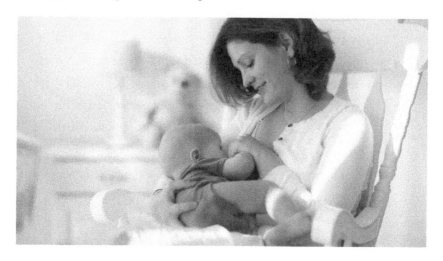

Sample morning routine for your 6- to 8-month-old baby

- Your baby wakes from a sleep. You decide whether to resettle her or if she's ready to get out of bed.
- If you decide it's time for her to get up, you greet her warmly and say hello.
- You change her nappy and start your social time together. Tell her what you're doing while you change her nappy and decide what sort of mood she's in. It's a good idea to tell her what sort of mood she's in as well. She doesn't know what she's feeling yet. She needs you to tell her that she's grumpy or happy or tired.
- You might decide she's hungry and ready for a milk feed, breakfast or lunch. When you feed her, have a routine so she knows she's going to have something to eat. Remember, when you have a meal, you always prepare yourself to eat.
- Tell her she's hungry and going to have a feed and what's she's going to have to eat – milk, banana, avocado. It's nice to know what type of food you're going to have for a meal.
- Talk to her while she's feeding – this is a social time. Just as you usually like to socialise and talk with someone when you have a meal, your baby really wants to enjoy your company during her meal and she'll eat better, too. (This is the time to put your phone away and use it later when she's asleep.)
- If you can, have something to eat at the same time. Eating together is always more comfortable and enjoyable.

- During her meal you can sing songs, tell stories and talk about the day so far and what you're going to do next. Talking, singing, smiling and gentle touching helps her brain grow and develop rapidly. Her language skills will develop more quickly.

- If she gets distracted, wait for her to have a break between sucks on the breast or bottle and then have a chat.

- Tell her when she's finished her milk or solids. She doesn't know yet when the meal is over, she needs you to tell her. By talking with her you are giving her cues and signals about what you are doing and what is about to happen.

- Clean her face and hands if she needs it and explain to her what you're doing. She needs a running commentary on everything that's happening to her. Most exciting of all, this will help your relationship to thrive. In the same way as any new and important relationship you have, the only way to get to know each other is to talk, socialise, smile and laugh.

- After her feed, she's probably ready for some play with you. When you play with her, she'll sometimes like to make up the game and invite you to help her. When she does that, follow her lead – that makes her feel confident and special. During this period, she might even have some solo play if she can keep her eye on you and this means you get to have a break.

- Watch for tired signs, which indicate when she's getting drowsy. Tell her she's tired and put her to bed using her usual bedtime routine.

Managing exciting activities at bedtime

Why is it that suddenly all the exciting activities start at bedtime? This is often dad time, isn't it? Dads are usually the ones with all those really fun games that wind everyone up. To be fair, mums do it too – but this is often the dad domain.

It's okay though, and perfectly normal, and why would anyone want to send in the fun police to stop something kids clearly love? In fact, 'dad games' provide a lot of important brain development. Dads play differently and no one wants to restrict such important play.

It's the aftermath and the fall-out that's often the problem. Because it's always when you want your baby, toddler or preschooler to go to bed, right?

The simple solution to this: don't expect your baby or child to go to bed straight after the fun. If the games are an unscheduled part of the routine, even though you or someone else might worry about them upsetting the plans for the evening, try not to let it become a source of frustration or a major family argument. Calculate it as part of the night-time routine and set a limit on it. You know it's going to happen anyway, so go with the flow and work it into your evening pattern.

For the first 12 months, your baby's capacity to tolerate play and stimulation is developing gradually, so you will need to learn her non-verbal language to understand when she's overstimulated, had enough of play and is ready for some quiet time prior to sleep. This is the time to start setting limits.

Toddlers and preschoolers manage longer periods of rough and tumble. You can tell them the game will soon be over and then it will be their bedtime routine.

At first, limits will be small and generally set for important reasons like safety. Setting small limits is helpful for both you and your child, because it can often be hard for both of you to stick to them. You have to be able to follow through and help your child with the limit you've set.

Children can be quite persistent in trying to accomplish a goal and they have far more energy than you. With that in mind, be sensitive and reasonable about limits, otherwise you'll spend your days in many exhausting and unwinnable battles. So it's always good to get your child used to the idea that there are small limits appropriate to her age.

As your child grows older and develops, limit-setting gets bigger. When you start with small, sensitive limits about important issues and work your way up, you and your child are used to the process of setting limits. It will be easier for you both. Bedtime games could be one of the first times you set a limit on yourself and your toddler.

When you plan your routine and set kind and reasonable limits, you can confidently handle the bedtime routine and feel in charge. This makes you feel good as a parent. Even though your toddler or preschooler might disagree with you about ending games, they don't know when enough is enough and need help to calm down. They're too little to make decisions about how excited they are. In the end, they'll be relieved not to have to make decisions or be in charge. Making adult decisions leaves them stressed and cranky.

After the games are over, the bedtime routine could start with a calming bath or shower. This is where you keep reminding your excited child that it's time to calm down for sleep and the bedtime routine begins. It will take about 30 minutes for her to calm down and relax, depending on her temperament and personality. Some children and adults get far more excited than others and take longer to settle and relax. You'll get to know what your child is like.

A very busy household

Busy households are a fact of life. When you first have your baby you may get some maternity leave, but you're still busy at home learning how to be a parent. First-time parents have a steep learning curve.

If you have two or more children, you are very busy managing several little people's needs, of different ages, all at once. Someone could need a sleep, someone could need a feed, someone could need to go to day care, preschool or school, and someone could need love and kisses all the time.

Homes need to be cleaned, meals need to be cooked, clothes cared for, bills paid and where's that social life and exercise that was mentioned somewhere?

Your life is busy enough when you stay at home, look after your baby and manage your home but, like many other parents, you may have to return to paid work or study sometime during the first 12 months of your baby's life. This often means having to use some type of child care. Life can become hectic and tiring.

Parents are by nature busy. You have a lot to do, such as:

- love and care for one or more children
- drop off and pick up children at child care or school
- drive a car or catch trains or buses to work or study
- manage your home, meals, bills and shopping
- find time for your partner, extended family and social life.

You can really have difficulty finding time for everything with so much going on. It's exhausting just reading this list!

But this is exactly how a very busy household can affect your baby/child's sleep. Now you could be thinking, 'Well, hold on a minute! I'm the one juggling all the work. Why does it affect my baby's sleep?'

Once again, think about the situation from your baby's or child's point of view. Often, your paid work or your study days start early.

Those mornings can be much busier and stressful than usual. You need to be organised if everyone is going to have breakfast and be dressed in time to get to child care and then your work or place of study. Your baby/child feels the difference in pace and will get to know the different routine means separation from you. This will mean some level of stress for her, no matter how much she enjoys child care or preschool. That's just normal.

A half or full day at child care can be exhausting for your baby or child. Think about it as their workplace. They are with their early childhood educators, some of whom they like and others not so much. They are spending their time with a group of babies or children, also some of whom they like and others they don't. Sometimes these groups are quite large and because your baby/child is still little, relationships can be difficult to manage without quite a bit of help.

Does it sound a bit similar to your own workplace? Instead of carers, you have a manager, and probably many co-worker relationships to navigate, which can be tiring.

Your baby or child will play throughout the day. Play is the business of childhood and is often underestimated in its importance. Babies and children work hard at play and are constantly learning and discovering.

All the time she is waiting for you to come and pick her up. She doesn't know how to tell the time, so she might, with your help, understand that you will arrive after a particular activity, such as afternoon tea. She really looks forward to you arriving, as what she wants most is to be with you.

After childcare pick-up, you arrive home tired but you still have heaps to do. You have to cook dinner, feed your baby, bathe her and put her to bed. Then there are household chores to do. Sometimes you might feel irritable and just want some time to yourself before your bedtime.

It's really easy to forget that your baby/child needs some wind-down time with you after child care. Busy households are like that. So what's the answer?

Babies and children work hard at play and are constantly learning and discovering.

Your baby/child has really missed you during the day and she's tired as well. She needs some special time with you as soon as you get home. That means adjusting your routine to include taking time out from cooking and cleaning for 30 to 45 minutes for a cuddle and a daily catch-up with your little one.

She needs to wind down and reconnect with you after such a long separation. This also provides her with stress relief from her busy day.

If she's old enough to talk, she needs you to ask questions about her day so you can find out what happened and whether it was a good or bad day. This allows you to celebrate her achievements and discover if something needs to be addressed with her carers. Additionally, when you give her this time as soon as you get home, she's more likely to settle into the evening and her bedtime routine without fussing and crying, which reduces the stress for everyone.

You will also benefit from sitting down and relaxing before starting your evening chores. Your evening routine may be set back 30 minutes or so, but you'll find it's worth it to have a more relaxed, less stressed baby/child. This will help you both sleep better.

Smartphones, tablets and TVs

In Chapter 1, there is an explanation of how blue light affects your baby's sleep (see page 6). Now that you have that information, you understand how important it is to remove electronic devices that emit blue light, such as televisions, smartphones, tablets and computers, from your baby's and/or child's sleep space. When you remove electronic devices, you will help establish your baby's circadian rhythm.

When you're developing a bedtime routine, you will probably like to include stories or sing songs. But this is definitely not the time for stories, songs or movies on smartphones, tablets or TVs, as that is far too stimulating at bedtime. This is the time for real books that your baby, toddler and preschooler can hold, touch, turn the pages and handle. She will enjoy pointing to the pictures and cuddling with you while you point to pictures or read. She will probably want you to read two to four stories.

Yes, it's a shame you have to put away the electronic devices because they're easy and you can find so many good programs that you know your child likes. But remember the end goal: sleep for both of you!

The games and programs aren't going anywhere – they'll be there for the times when you and your baby or children are not going to bed.

Going on holidays

Another sleep environment and bedtime routine you need to consider is when you decide to go on a holiday with your baby or child. Whenever you go away, you'll need to adjust your baby's sleep environment and bedtime routine to a new one.

Holidays with children are different, there's no getting away from that fact. If you try to have the same types of relaxing getaways you had before having a baby, you'll be really stressed and disappointed.

Travelling with your child means you will need to:
- do lots of planning beforehand
- take quite a bit of extra luggage
- make your holiday simple, child-oriented and fun
- take a little longer to get where you're going
- explain to your child what a holiday is and prepare her for the travel as well as the fun.

If you do all that, you'll enjoy your holiday more and be a lot less stressed. There's nothing worse than a bored toddler or preschooler running riot while you try to be thrilled by the Grand Canyon or visit a museum. Even a museum with dinosaurs will only interest your little one for 5 or 10 minutes.

Your child has a short attention span and can't cope with too many grown-up adventures or a holiday chock-a-block with sightseeing tours. If you're unsure about where to go for a holiday with her, start with an internet search or ask a travel agent to find out what's available and suitable for a family holiday with very young children.

Once you've made the decision about where to go, you'll need to choose your accommodation. If you're not going to stay with friends or family, then finding a hotel with self-contained apartments is probably the most comfortable option for you. That way you can have cooking facilities, a small living area and an extra bedroom. You won't regret this choice. You'll have somewhere separate to put your child to bed and space for you. Some hotels may also have babysitting facilities so you can have a break, but check the prices.

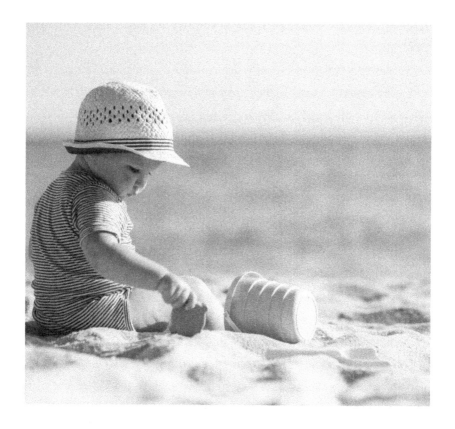

Travelling by car

Whenever you travel by car, make sure you have the correct baby capsule or car seat for her age, and ensure it is fitted properly. You will probably need a shade visor on the windows to reduce the sun and the heat off your little one during the drive. Please refer to additional information about car safety in Chapter 1: How sleep works, on pages 15–16.

When you drive with young children, you need to be prepared to make plenty of stops for play breaks, nappy changes, soothing and feeding. If your child gets motion sickness, you will have to make frequent stops for that, too. Speak to your doctor about how to manage car trips.

How often you stop is really determined by your child's needs, but it may be every 2 hours. Make sure you have some toys to rotate, plenty of water in spill-proof bottles and some favourite snacks. If your child needs a dummy or comforter, have that on hand.

Some children will sleep in the car while you're driving but wake up as soon as you stop. This can work to your advantage because it enables you to get to your destination more quickly. But if your little one sleeps too much in the car, she may take longer to go to sleep in the evening. If she just takes her usual naps in the car, you may be able to keep her to her usual routine, but she will still be excited and more difficult to settle in her new surroundings.

Travelling by plane

If you travel by plane, try to catch an overnight flight so your little one can stay with her night-time sleep routine. Once your toddler is 2 years old, you will have to book her a seat on an international flight. If you have a young baby, you can ask for a bassinet when you book your seat. The bassinet seats have a lot of floor room, so if you have a toddler, these are good seats to book.

Establishing routines on holiday

Once you've arrived and settled in at your holiday destination, let your child explore the accommodation and get her bearings. She'll want to look at where you'll be sleeping and also where she'll be sleeping. This is very important to her because she needs to feel safe when she's asleep. Remember, you're all sleeping in a strange, new place a long way from home. She has to be sure she knows where you are if she needs you, so give her time to look around.

No matter where you are in the world, you're going to want to keep her in a routine. This is not so bad if your time change isn't more than an hour or two. But if you cross more than three time zones, then you and your child will experience jet lag. This simply means that the travel messes up your circadian rhythms which are set to the time zone you live in (see Chapter 1: How sleep works).

Managing jet lag

To manage your child's sleep during a jet-lagged, unsettled period, follow these suggestions:
- Maintain a predictable yet flexible daily routine.
- Help your child get used to eating meals when she would usually be asleep by keeping meal times to local hours and give her small meals with little snacks.
- Ensure you maintain your soothing, relaxing bedtime routine.
- Use the age-related settling strategies in chapters 7 and 8 to help her fall asleep and resettle if she wakes through the night.
- Wake your child in the morning, even if she's had trouble falling asleep and had a late night.

It takes about a week to adjust to a destination that crosses three or more time zones – such as Sydney to Los Angeles. During this period, while you reset your child's circadian clock to the new time zone, she will be unsettled and often irritable. When you fly home, you will go through the process again.

If your travel involves a time change of only an hour or two, then keeping to her routine will be much easier to manage. You have two choices:

1. Adjust to the small difference in time and try to work around local time. This would mean your routines, meals and bedtime would be 1 to 2 hours earlier or later than at home, which may be tricky depending on the age of your child.
2. Stay with your regular home hours for the duration of your holiday. This strategy will also make things easier once you return home.

Whatever you decide to do, try and maintain the predictability of your child's daily routines and bedtime routines as closely as you can. This means planning your day's activities around meals and naps, and having some busy days with down-time days in between where you all rest and relax. If you have a toddler or preschooler, she may not get a proper nap every day when you're on holiday; when she can't have a nap, you need to set aside some quiet time or a break for her.

Finally, when you travel, you need to always be prepared for anything. In particular, think about what your child likes to eat, because the food at your destination may not suit her. It's easy to think, 'I won't bother taking that, I'll buy it when I get there.' But you might get a horrible shock if the product you and your child desperately need doesn't exist at your destination. Always take important stuff with you.

Make yourself a list of important items to take, for example:

- appropriate cot and bedding for your child if the hotel, apartment or house you're staying at doesn't have them
- prams, capsules, sunhat
- comforter, dummy and spares, any special bedding
- clothes, nappies, baby wipes, creams and nappy bags
- some favourite toys
- special foods, favourite snacks
- milk/formula and spill-proof drink bottles
- first-aid kit, thermometer, sunscreen and any medication your child needs.

Let's face it, holidays with your child aren't the relaxing getaways you used to have. That's why families with young children often end up taking a short drive or plane trip to have a fun beach holiday. After all, it's just a giant sandpit with lots of water nearby to splash in, so it may be the easiest holiday of all.

With a little online research, precision organising, expert packing and the expectation that this holiday will be fun, you will enjoy a trip away with your little one.

In this chapter, we looked at the types of obstacles in your environment that can affect your baby's sleep and how you can make your baby's environment more conducive to sleep. Many of these obstacles are old habits or routines that you may not have thought much about. Going on holidays is something new to consider when you think about sleep environments and that takes a lot of planning and organising. However, once you start thinking them through and with some careful planning and support from your partner and family, you can change, manage or eliminate the obstacles in your environment and create a routine that meets the needs of you and your baby.

Christina's story (mother of Zac, 13 months)

Zac was a wakeful baby from the very beginning. Even in the hospital, all the other babies in the nursery would be sleeping soundly and he was awake and taking in his surroundings or crying. I knew I wouldn't get too much sleep in the early days, but it was ridiculous. During the day he would wake after 20 minutes and he was up six to eight times at night.

It was after I started mothers' group that I realised his sleep behaviour was pretty different to the other babies'. The paediatrician recommended some medication as it was suspected my little guy was suffering from reflux. This did improve things a bit – he started sleeping slightly longer during the day and at night only woke three or four times (on a good night). It was far from ideal, though.

I went to the Early Childhood Centre and they told me to use white noise for his sleeps to help him transition from one cycle to another. They also recommended darkening his room a bit when he was having his day sleeps. I don't think these things really helped at the time but they're great now, as he doesn't wake when the sun comes up in the mornings.

When he was around 6 months, an early childhood nurse told us to get him into a routine. The nurse told us he had to have one sleep a day in his cot with the white noise. It always had to be the same sleep each day, to ensure he got used to it. We also started a bedtime routine to get him to sleep at night. I would give him dinner, then his bath, a milk feed, then we'd read him a book. We'd always sing 'Twinkle Twinkle Little Star' to him before he went to sleep.

He was still not sleeping for very long during the day but the routine really helped him learn to self-settle. I no longer had to lie in there patting his tummy or the cot mattress, I would just put him in bed and he would go to sleep quickly.

I think the big change to the length of his naps and night sleeps was when he started to walk at around 10 months. It was like he was starting to wear himself out and within a week or two, he was doing 2-hour naps during the day and sleeping through most nights.

I think with my little guy, he just found the world too big and exciting to waste time napping. However, the routines really helped, as I think he realised that it all went in a cycle. If he was put down to bed the same way, then the world would still be there to explore when he woke up.

Key message

- Your baby needs her own safe, comfy room and bed. She also needs to be put to sleep in the same bed and room for her day and night sleeps. This will help her night-time sleep.
- If you choose to move your baby to her own room between 6 and 12 months, she may learn to self-settle more quickly when she wakes at night. This is because you're less likely to hear her when she rouses and calls you.
- Having familiar daily routines will provide your baby with a predictable and stress-free atmosphere during the day, which will prepare her for the night and sleep.
- Going on holidays requires you to think about your baby/child's sleep environment and routines in a different way. You will need to do lots of preparation and organisation so all of you can have a relaxing and fun holiday together.

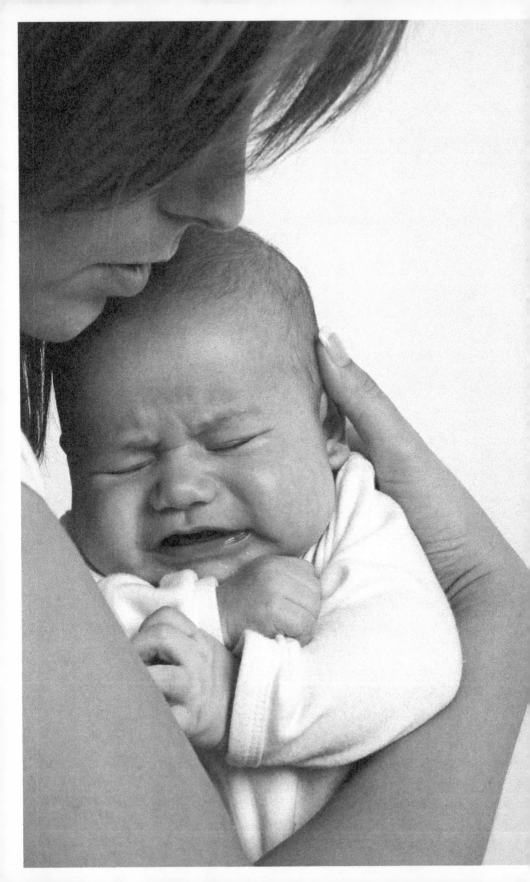

CHAPTER 5

Why your baby cries

The most common cause for your baby crying, particularly during the first three months, is to alert you that she needs to re-establish and maintain close physical contact with you. This type of crying is an instinctive need and has a very important function, quite separate from her physical needs.

Crying to maintain close physical contact with you is a social and emotional need. Social and emotional development is one of the most important developmental tasks of the first three years of life.

Your baby can't physically follow you around yet, so she cries to keep you close to her. She needs your presence to feel safe and secure. When she can't see you, she doesn't know where you are, so she will fuss and cry. If you don't appear soon enough, she will give you a stronger signal that she really needs you and cry more persistently.

When you respond promptly by going to her with love, reassurance and affection, you make her feel safe and secure. This is how she forms her attachment to you. She cries and calls; you respond with reassurance and help; she feels happy and safe, able to relax and enjoy a feed, social time or sleep.

That's how your social and emotional relationship with each other develops – and that's how your baby's attachment to you forms. This bonding is also vital in helping your baby's brain to grow and develop in a healthy way.

Research shows that babies cry more when they are separated from their parents and calm once they're physically back together again. Humans have evolved to carry their babies to ensure survival from predators, as infants cannot run away from danger on their own.

This means that when your baby is separated from you and begins to miss you, she will cry out for you. This type of call for attention and help is a normal response to a physical or emotional need.

Her physical need means she fusses and cries for comfort for a range of reasons, including help with:

- a nappy change
- a feed
- a sleep
- a physical complaint, like a tummy upset
- feeling uncomfortable, like hot or cold.

An emotional need means your baby needs you to help her to manage feelings of:

- loneliness
- anger
- sadness
- fear
- overstimulation
- happiness and joy.

Your baby needs to be close to you so you can help her manage all the strange and new physical and emotional experiences she has to cope with. Having so many new feelings and experiences is exhausting for her. She can't manage them without your help, so she cries for you. Her crying is a powerful signal to you. The pitch of her cry triggers a physical and psychological stress reaction in you, which helps you to intuitively go to your baby to soothe and help her. This type of stress activation comes from your evolutionary roots and drives your response to your baby. Your baby's cry is supposed to cause you some stress – if it didn't, you probably wouldn't respond.

Parents have always used body contact, facial and eye contact, a soothing singsong voice and rocking to help their crying baby. In return, your baby calms and usually snuggles close. This gives you confidence that you can help her and you both feel satisfied and enjoy your relationship more.

People used to think you could tell by your baby's cry when she was hungry, tired or in pain, but it's now understood you cannot distinguish a hunger cry from a tired cry or a bored cry. However, you can tell what your baby needs from the degree and pitch of her cry, together with what her non-verbal language is indicating to you.

You can work out how urgent your baby's cry is but not what's causing it. The most important thing to do is carefully listen to her, observe her and get to know her non-verbal language. The more experienced you become with observing your baby's cues and responding promptly when she cries, the better you'll understand what she's trying to tell you (see Chapter 6: How your baby communicates).

In the first three months, crying is the best way she has to communicate with you. When she's older, she will begin to find other ways to communicate. And that's when you find her crying communicates definite needs – for example, you can see she's frightened of a stranger and needs your comfort. But until she can physically follow you to stay close or verbally say what she needs, crying will always be her first and best way to tell you she needs to be close to gain comfort and safety.

Generally, the quicker you attend to your baby's crying, the quicker she will stop crying and calm down again. Responding quickly and sensitively to your baby each time she cries is thought to help reduce the overall amount of crying she does. The slower you respond to your crying baby, the more she cries and the longer it takes for you to calm her down.

You can expect your child to continue to need your safety and reassurance when she's upset right through the first three years. This is not spoiling her; in fact, you have exactly the same needs when you're upset.

When something upsetting happens, it's common to contact your family or close friends and cry or confide your problems. When you do that, you're seeking safety and reassurance. If you don't receive the comfort you're seeking it feels awful.

Your baby is just the same as you. She needs comfort and reassurance when she cries. When she gets that, it helps her to develop an understanding that when she asks for help she will get it.

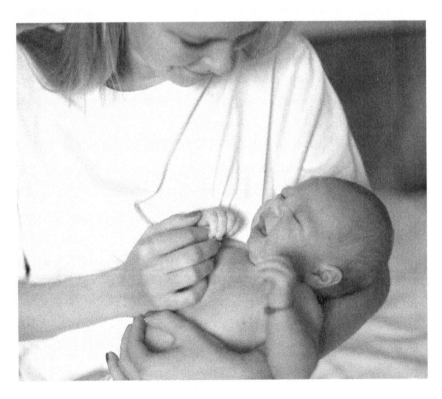

When you can't soothe your baby

Unfortunately, there will be times during the first three months when you can't soothe your baby, and she may continue to cry no matter what you try to do. This sort of crying is a part of what's called 'normal developmental crying'.

Your baby's crying usually follows developmental patterns. Normal developmental crying usually starts to increase at 2 weeks after birth and continues to build up to a peak when she's around 2 months old. Crying then starts to taper off again, and by 3 to 4 months old, her crying will be less frequent.

During this normal developmental crying phase, you may notice that your baby has bouts of intense, inconsolable crying in the afternoons and evenings. You often really notice this type of crying during the second month or at the peak stage of the normal crying period, around 6 weeks.

You probably want to know how long will your baby cry. Each baby is an individual and some cry for longer than others. Your baby could cry as little as 1 hour per day or as much as 5 hours per day.

The slower you respond to your crying baby, the more she cries and the longer it takes for you to calm her down.

Both lengths of crying are within a normal range. However, 5 hours of crying is very hard for you to manage. Sometimes this type of crying is called 'colic' – but it's still part of normal developmental crying and will usually resolve by 3 to 4 months of age.

There are some popular and traditional reasons that could influence the ways you might be thinking about your baby's crying, such as these possible reasons:

- She's being manipulative.
- She's looking for attention.
- She's being a 'drama queen'.
- When you attend to your baby during the day and night you are reinforcing 'attention-seeking' behaviour.
- You'll spoil your baby by giving her too much attention.
- You're making her too dependent on you.
- You're weak if you 'give in' to her.

None of these reasons is true, of course. The early-20th century behavioural psychologist John B. Watson came up with ideas about disciplining and training babies and children. He believed you could condition a baby to stop crying by ignoring her. Unfortunately, other 'childcare experts' over the years have continued to promote his ideas.

Respond to your baby's crying

A good example of conditioning a baby to stop crying by not responding until she gives up crying is called 'controlled crying'. But evolution intended parents to respond to their baby's cry in the early years of a child's life.

Today's knowledge about your baby's early brain and social and emotional development has shown that these old ideas about ignoring your baby's emotional and social needs actually interfere with a critical period of her early brain development. These ideas also interfere with the development of your baby's very important first relationship with you.

Consider her first relationship with you as her first experience of falling in love. She wants to be with you, gaze into your eyes, cuddle with you and talk to you. She's learning what love feels like. Remember what it feels like to fall in love?

Your baby is and has to be dependent on you and will be for a long time. She needs lots of warmth and caring attention, especially during this early period.

So, this early stage of crying is her way of telling you she needs you. She just wants to be with you, which is normal. If she didn't seek your attention, she wouldn't survive. When you think about it like that, crying isn't bad – crying is healthy, necessary and a good thing.

During the first 12 months, your baby is supposed to seek your attention, she is supposed to be dependent on you and needs to be responded to while she's young and vulnerable. When you attend to her crying, you aren't reinforcing her to cry. You are soothing her, empathising with and reassuring her, just the same as someone soothes and reassures you when you cry.

If someone comforts and soothes you when you're upset and crying, you tend to calm down and relax more quickly and feel better. You're able to get on with your day more easily. And the opposite is also true. If you have a long cry and no one is there to comfort you, you often feel exhausted and sad at the end of it. A worse scenario is, if you are very upset and cry and someone you love is there but they ignore you. You feel rejected, hurt and confused.

Your baby is the same. Once you've soothed and comforted her, she's more able to play and socialise and get on with her day. Everyone likes to feel comforted and understood.

Excessive crying

Babies who cry excessively are the ones at the extreme upper end of the normal range of crying 1 to 5 hours per day.

How can you tell if your baby is crying excessively and you both need extra help and support? Well, if your baby is otherwise well and healthy, and she displays the following three behaviours, then her crying is moving outside the normal range and towards excessive. She cries and fusses for more than:

- three hours a day
- three days a week
- three weeks.

This type of excessive crying is often long, drawn out and persistent, and your baby seems to be inconsolable. During these bouts of crying it seems that nothing you do can help her to calm down.

Some of the behaviours you might notice are, she:

- resists being held
- resists being laid down
- resists being cuddled and won't snuggle in for comfort
- becomes stiff and arches her back
- prefers to be held upright
- looks wide-eyed and frightened
- needs you to rock, sway, nurse and walk with her for hours at a time
- doesn't want to look at you
- doesn't seem to be able to shut down or fights against falling asleep
- sometimes has a swollen tummy and flexed knees, which makes you think she has wind or colic
- cluster feeds towards late afternoon and evening.

This type of crying is due to immature neurobiological processes that occur during the first 3 to 4 months. At about 3 months, your baby will have a major developmental growth change and the crying usually resolves by 4 months.

Knowing that this sort of crying is normal and there's nothing wrong with your baby can be reassuring. The crying will reduce. It's also good to know that just because your baby may cry excessively during the first 3 to 4 months, it doesn't always mean that she'll be more wakeful and fuss and cry at night after these first few months. After normal developmental crying resolves at around 3 to 4 months, her sleep and settling patterns will continue to mature as normal and average crying per day will be about 1 hour.

If you are worried there might be something medically wrong with your baby, such as colic, gastro-oesophageal reflux or some other illness, visit your child and family health nurse or your family doctor for help and advice. They can guide you on further steps to take.

You can also look in Chapter 12: Common illnesses and other sleep disruptions, for a description of common problems, such as colic and gastro-oesophageal reflux (GOR), that can cause crying.

Coping with your baby's crying

Excessive amounts of crying – 3 hours or more a day – are difficult to manage continuously. That's when you begin to doubt yourself. You can also become so exhausted and focused on the difficulties of the crying that you begin to miss those times of the day when your baby is not crying, such as when she's quiet and ready to socialise or play briefly, often in the morning.

Unfortunately, your baby's excessive, prolonged and unsoothable crying can have an intense emotional effect on you and it may become harder to respond to your baby in a calm way. You can begin to feel:

- constantly exhausted
- overloaded
- helpless
- fearful
- on edge and alarmed
- angry or aggressive
- guilty for feeling angry or aggressive
- a sense of failure as a good parent
- powerless at being unable to help your baby
- lowered self-esteem
- a loss of confidence.

And if you are anxious or depressed, the crying may seem even worse for you.

When your baby consistently has excessive and prolonged bouts of crying, your usual sensitive and soothing responses may not seem to work and you can feel disorganised and desperate in the way that you respond to her.

The following scenario is an example of excessive crying and is thought to occur for 16 to 20 per cent of babies and their parents:

Scenario: excessive crying

During the first two to three weeks after birth, your baby may have only cried when she was hungry, grumpy or tired. Soothing her was easier and you usually fed her, changed her or just picked her up, rocked, patted or sang to her and she snuggled in and calmed down. You would both have felt satisfied and continued to feel satisfied each time that happened. Feeding and social interactions were more enjoyable when she wasn't crying because you knew you could soothe her. You and your baby's relationship was in a positive feedback loop – that is, you did something positive and she did something positive in return. When that kept happening, you both enjoyed and felt satisfied with your relationship.

At 3 weeks old, the routine started to change as her normal developmental crying phase began. Her crying slowly increased and she wasn't as easy to soothe. You didn't understand what was happening and you thought something might be wrong with her.

By 6 weeks old, she was crying for 3½ hours every evening and there was nothing you could do to stop her. She arched her back, screamed and looked like she was in pain. She didn't want you to put her down but didn't seem like she wanted you to hold her either. All she wanted was for you to walk around with her. Her crying was unpredictable, there was no explanation for it and you never knew how long it was going to last. You didn't expect having a baby to be like this.

Your partner and mother couldn't soothe her either and you felt like everyone was blaming you. You blamed yourself. Everyone seemed to have a reason why your baby was crying but no one had an answer. You fearfully started to anticipate the crying episodes.

You didn't think your baby liked you anymore. You cried and felt helpless, overwhelmed, angry and guilty. Sometimes you just couldn't go to her when she cried and so you left her to cry while you calmed yourself a bit, but this made you feel like a failure.

You or your partner drove her around in the car to get her to sleep. When she finally fell asleep at midnight, you felt shattered and exhausted. Feeding her was often difficult and social times weren't enjoyable either.

You and your baby's relationship had become a negative feedback loop and unsatisfying.

Excessive crying will create intense and conflicting emotional effects inside you, such as anxiety, an urge to comfort and calm your baby, an urge to run away, fear, increasing frustration, anger, love and warmth. This is a very exhausting and confusing time for you.

Excessive infant crying can lead to:
- problems in your relationship with your baby that can contribute to persistent crying
- postnatal depression and/or anxiety
- relationship difficulties with your partner or family
- shaken baby syndrome.

What you can do

First and most importantly, remember that your baby is not crying because of:

- your lack of care and effort to soothe her
- your inexperience
- her birth order
- having a difficult temperament.

You must reassure yourself that it's not your fault that your baby is crying. You also need to find someone you can talk to who will listen to you and support you.

Don't try and tough it out on your own, without someone to help you with all those intense feelings, fears and worries that something might be wrong with you and your baby. If you are concerned about your baby, you can visit your local child and family health nurse, who will check her and be able to reassure you that there is nothing physically wrong. On the rare occasion that a health need is identified, your nurse will be able to refer you to the appropriate health professional.

This 'someone' you reach out to mustn't undermine your confidence any further. If you feel like you're being undermined and feel blamed by someone you're seeking help from, then don't keep speaking to that person, find someone else.

You're having a hard time and you deserve to be supported, listened to and helped. This is not the time for lecturing or blaming. You and your baby need comfort and care during this difficult period.

When supporting your baby through this time, the first thing to attend to is her day–night sleep rhythms (see chapters 1 to 3). Next is to make sure you have a predictable daily and bedtime routine in place (see Chapter 4: Creating a conducive sleep environment). A predictable daily routine will keep her more relaxed.

It's also important to be able to recognise her non-verbal body language. She will signal to you when she's had enough interaction with you or there's too much stimulation in her environment. A baby who cries excessively probably can't cope with being overstimulated, so you will need to avoid that happening.

Recognise, too, when she's getting tired and ready to sleep. In the first three months, your baby should tire and be ready for sleep about 1 to 1½ hours after her last sleep. If your baby cries excessively, stay very alert for signs of drowsiness so she doesn't get overstimulated and over-alert. In Chapter 6: How your baby communicates, you'll learn more about understanding your baby's non-verbal language.

When you are playing and socialising with your baby, go for relaxing types of play rather than vigorous, very stimulating play. Her play periods may be quite brief, so make sure she's ready and interested in talking and playing and watch for signs when she's had enough.

The sorts of signs she'll give when she's had enough are:

- looking away
- looking down
- pushing the toy away
- having glazed or droopy eyes
- fussing
- kicking.

When she's doing any of these, just sit back and wait to see what she does next. This behaviour may mean playtime is over. She'll look back at you if she wants to play some more.

If she keeps fussing and moving her arms and legs in all different directions, this is a sign that it's no longer time to play and socialise. Continuing will only overstimulate her and lead to full-blown crying, so she now needs calm and soothing actions from you.

The most effective method to soothe a crying baby is to carry her.

Soothing actions for your crying baby

There are lots of ways to soothe a crying baby. In fact, there are an overwhelming number of methods available in books and on the internet. There are crying baby apps, white noise apps, baby sleep sounds apps, massage oils, music, swings, baby slings, changing baby formula and prescription medicines.

But what methods work? Well, the effectiveness of these methods has been hard to measure or prove because most babies start their normal developmental crying at around 2 to 3 weeks and by 3 to 4 months their crying resolves anyway.

That can mean that each of these methods to stop your baby crying seems to work because you bought equipment or used a method at the peak of her crying at 6 weeks and after a week or so it worked. At the same time, your baby's crying is going to start decreasing and resolve at 3 to 4 months by itself. That's why no one has proved that the methods do or don't work. Any of these methods are perfectly fine if they work for you and you have checked that the equipment is safe for your baby's developmental stage.

'Well that's no good to me!' you say. And you're right.

The most effective method to soothe a crying baby is to carry her. Most studies have found increased carrying reduces crying. If your baby cries excessively you're probably already carrying her most of the day, so let's look at some other ideas.

Soothing strategies to reduce crying

It's important to use a range of three or four gentle and affectionate strategies that are easy to follow and have a slow, soothing pace. These examples might suit you and your baby:

- Carry her in a sling next to your chest, making sure you're as relaxed as you can be. She will be able to hear your heartbeat, so you won't need a heartbeat app.
- Speak to her in a calm, soothing voice.
- Sing to her in a soft, low voice.
- Cuddle her.
- Put her on her back or tummy and use a gentle pat, rub or touch to soothe her.
- Take her for a walk in her pram.
- When she's very upset and crying, place her in a firm wrap or just gently hold her arms and hands.
- If you use white noise, baby-safe massage oil, etc., then incorporate that into your soothing routine.

Whatever strategy you decide to use, don't keep changing it for new and different ones recommended to you by friends, family or the internet. Stick with the soothing and calming strategies you feel comfortable with and make them part of your routine.

Your baby needs familiarity with your soothing strategy so she can relax and not be overstimulated with too much variety and change. Remaining calm, consistent and predictable is really important to her.

When your baby is ready for sleep, she needs to be firmly but comfortably wrapped in a soft wrap, with her arms flexed against her chest so she can get her hands to her mouth in case she wants to suck them, to prevent her from startling herself and then overstimulating herself. She may appear to struggle initially but most babies will respond to the feeling of being wrapped as it gives a sense of being contained, safe and secure.

If you feel very distressed, anxious, angry or aggressive because your attempts to soothe your baby aren't working, put your baby in a safe place, such as her cot or crib, and take a break. It's perfectly fine for you to walk away and take some time to calm down. This is the best thing for you and your baby, and it doesn't mean you're a bad parent. What it means is that you need some help, rest and support. You could contact Tresillian's live advice website or ring the parent helpline (see page 276) for support and guidance in those moments.

By 3 to 4 months of age, most babies will have resolved this crying period with no long-term negative effects. About 5 per cent of babies continue to be unsettled at 5 months. If your baby continues to be unsettled and cry for long periods, seek advice from a health professional to ensure she is physically well.

You will also need to ensure you have adequate emotional support. Coping with a crying baby for five months will put a strain on your close relationships, including with your baby. The support of your family and friends isn't always enough, because they don't always understand all the intense feelings you might be experiencing.

Talking to your child and family health nurse or a counsellor, such as a social worker or psychologist, who works with parents and babies, may give you some much-needed space where you can offload your pent-up feelings. Talking therapy can help you and your baby enjoy each other again.

If you feel very distressed, anxious, angry
or aggressive because your attempts
to soothe your baby aren't working,
put your baby in a safe place, such as
her cot or crib, and take a break.

Shaken Baby Syndrome

This is a form of injury to a baby caused by violent shaking, an impact to the baby's head or both. When a baby is violently shaken out of frustration or anger by an adult, her heavy head jerks back and forwards on her weak neck. This makes her brain move about in her skull and it gets injured. Shaking a baby can cause serious brain damage, which can lead to mental retardation, learning deficits and behavioural problems. Ultimately, it can cause death.

This injury usually happens because a parent or other caregiver loses control of their emotions. They usually don't mean to, but they can become so frustrated and angry with the baby's crying that they pick her up and forcefully shake her to make her stop.

Evidence indicates excessive infant crying is the most common cause of Shaken Baby Syndrome. Shaking a baby does stop crying, but that's because the baby has experienced a blow to the head similar to a concussion injury.

Much of this heightened frustration and anger can come from a parent feeling that they are unable to calm their baby and meet their baby's needs, or from a caregiver wanting to stop the crying.

For more information on Shaken Baby Syndrome and ways to manage prolonged crying, visit the Purple Crying website and Kids Health website (see page 279).

After 3 months

At about 3 months of age, your baby undergoes a major developmental change and becomes more socially aware. This is when her non-specific type of crying resolves. At this age, her crying starts to become more purposeful and social. Her crying will usually be directed at someone and her preference is you. After 6 months, she will definitely prefer her favourite person above anyone else. However, after 3 months you still need to respond to her crying in just the same way you have been doing. She still needs your soothing and loving response when she's upset.

After she is through her peak crying period, your baby will definitely be signalling and trying to communicate with you through both vocalisations and crying. If you have been responding predictably and promptly to her cries through the early months, she will anticipate your soothing actions and begin to quiet when she sees you, sometimes even before you give her physical contact.

This is how your baby learns that her communications mean something and are a way to gain your help to achieve a goal. Asking for help is important for all future learning. This enables her to know that it's all right to ask for help when she has problems later in life, such as when she's at school.

At 6 months, your baby can use her crying to protest about something she doesn't like, such as getting her nose wiped. Protest crying continues well into the second year. It's normal for her to protest about something she doesn't like and crying is the way she will tell you. You need to remain calm and soothing as you continue to wipe her nose or wash her face so she knows everything is okay.

By 6 months, you are her most favourite person in the whole world and she misses you when you're not around, so she'll cry and call to you. This behaviour is usually called 'separation anxiety', and it happens to all babies between 6 to 8 months. She cries because she doesn't know where you are, or if you're going to come back. Her brain isn't mature enough to know that yet.

Eventually, she will learn that each time you leave a room, or leave her to go to sleep, or at day care, you will return. At the same time, she's going to cry when you separate from her – a separation cry. Each time you come back from a separation, she needs you to gently reassure her. You use the same familiar soothing strategies you've developed over the first three to six months. You continue to soothe her until she's calm and ready to play, go back to sleep or return to whatever the present activity might be.

After a while she'll understand and trust that you'll come back to her. But many children will still suffer from separation anxiety right into their third year. When it resolves will depend on many factors, including her temperament and personality.

When your baby is 9 months old, she will go through another major developmental growth period. Her brain is growing rapidly and her

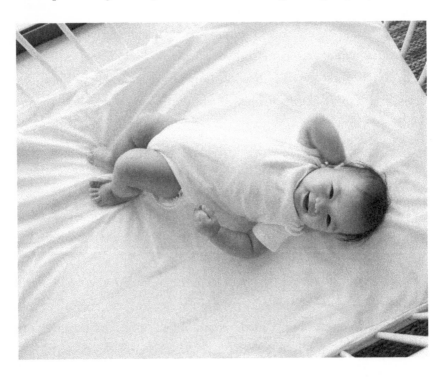

social and emotional development is maturing along with it. She shows great interest in other people and wants to gain much more of your social attention. This is the time when your baby becomes much more sociable and interested in what's going on around her.

From nine months onwards, your baby uses crying to let you know that she has a physical, emotional or social discomfort that she needs you to help her with. She uses her cry as a clear communication of her need to get your attention. When she cries, she will look at you in her effort to communicate with you. She usually accompanies her crying by holding out her arms to you, clinging to you and crawling to you if she's able.

The types of physical needs that make her cry remain the same. She cries because she needs something to eat, a nappy change, needs to sleep or she might have hurt herself. At this age, she has clear social and emotional needs, such as a fear of strangers or animals. She can protest cry at an older sibling who is bothering her, or she may be lonely for your company.

This is when your baby is becoming very much part of the family and a sociable person in her own right. She wants to be involved with family goings-on.

It's also when another peak of crying occurs, but this time it's at night. Once again, there's nothing wrong with her, she is going through a normal developmental phase. This crying can signal further sleep problems if you don't put into place a bedtime routine and some gentle, reassuring sleep and settling strategies.

What you can do

Crying at this age has a much more social component, so as well as the soothing routine you've already established, you can try other ways of responding to your baby. First of all, determine whether she has a physical need or a social need.

Crying for physical needs can be met easily with a feed, sleep, nappy change or attention to sickness or pain. You would respond to her cries in the same way you have done through the previous three months – promptly, gently and with some sort of soothing action.

You can respond to your baby's social crying initially by speaking to her and showing her your face to reassure her. Sometimes singing, rocking or even distraction with a game can work. If she is very upset, just as you did when she was younger, use some sort of gentle physical touch to soothe her. Physical contact usually stops crying more quickly than anything else.

Whatever the reason your baby cries, make sure you respond to her as promptly as possible so she doesn't get too upset. The more upset she is, the longer it will take her to calm down.

Crying is your baby's best way of communicating with you in the first three to four months of her life. She cries because she wants to be close to you, especially when she's tired, lonely, hungry or just needs a cuddle. During her first 3 to 4 months, she will go through a normal developmental crying stage. During this period, her crying will increase and at about 6 to 8 weeks she might cry as much as 3 to 4 hours a day. This can be very hard for you to manage, but it's important to remember that she will stop crying. By 3 to 4 months, she will find lots of other ways to communicate with you and her crying will reduce.

All babies have periods of crying when you can't soothe them – remember, it's not because you're a bad parent or that you're doing something wrong. As long as you try to comfort and reassure your baby that you're there to help, she'll soon learn that she can rely on you to help her when she's upset.

If your baby does cry a lot and it's getting you down, try to get support from your family, friends and/or a health professional to make sure that you remain emotionally and physically well so you can continue to provide the care and attention that you want to give to your baby.

Alison's story (mother of Jack, 6 months)

I found the first few months of my son's life really tough. For the first 12 weeks he just cried and cried. He wouldn't sleep unless he was in my arms, so I would sit up in bed holding him all night long.

We were going to see the early childhood nurse every week as he wasn't putting on weight and she referred us to Tresillian. She said I was bordering on postnatal depression. To be honest, I think my issues with my son started well before he was born.

We struggled for almost four years to conceive and went through countless rounds of IVF. When we finally found out we were pregnant, we were thrilled of course, but then reality set in. I was pretty anxious about my pregnancy, and we were worried about money and how we were going to cope with a small baby. I went to see the midwives at the hospital and they referred me to a psychologist who said I was suffering antenatal anxiety.

By the time little Jack arrived, I was already pretty worn out but things just got worse. He was crying a lot and because he wasn't putting on weight, I thought he was hungry so I tried to feed him all the time. He was probably crying out of tiredness but I wasn't very confident and just didn't know what to do.

The nurses at Tresillian gave me so much confidence in tackling the sleeping issues by showing me how to look for his tired signs (Jack gets really jerky when he's tired) and then how to settle him in my arms until he was relaxed and drowsy. I then learned to put him down in his cot and pat him gently while saying 'shhh' until he was asleep.

We also tackled the feeding issues. We started with one tactic that didn't work as he kept losing weight, so we tried another that worked much better. For every second breastfeed, I would pump what I had left, then give it to him as a top-up after the following feed. They even let me remain in the Residential Stay for a few extra nights to make sure it was all working, which I really appreciated.

When I got home, it was like I had a different baby. For the very first nap I put him down in his cot, used the techniques I'd learned and he went right to sleep! For the first week I needed to pat him to sleep, but after that it was like something clicked and he started to go to sleep on his own. These days he prefers to self-settle, it's amazing!

Sometimes I feel sad when I see newborn babies as I feel like I missed out on really enjoying that stage. But I'm so glad I got help when I did, and I wouldn't hesitate to go back if I needed help in the future.

Key message

- Today's knowledge about your baby's early brain and social and emotional development has shown that the old ideas about ignoring your baby's emotional and social needs actually interfere with a critical period of her early brain development.
- You must reassure yourself that it's not your fault that your baby is crying. You also need to find someone you can talk to who will listen to you and support you.
- Whatever the reason your baby cries, respond to her promptly and sensitively, and follow a predictable, soothing routine.

CHAPTER 6

How your baby communicates

Right from birth your baby is spellbound by human faces, especially yours. This preference for looking at faces is believed to be hardwired into our brain.

The first thing your baby will want to do when she's born is look at your face, gaze into your eyes, grasp your finger with her tiny hand and snuggle in close to you. Her body language gives you a powerful message of, 'Hello! I want to know you. I'm so glad to be with you at last.'

This is one of the first times you experience your baby's amazing ability to communicate with you through non-verbal language. When you gaze back at her you feel a rush of 'love hormones' that help you to connect and know each other. Sometimes this doesn't happen immediately, but it will eventually.

After you both enjoy your first meeting, you have your first breastfeed or formula feed together. Everyone always says hello and has a chat before they have a meal together.

Non-verbal cues

Your baby can't communicate her needs to you with words until well into her second year, and even then she will have some trouble communicating all her needs with words. But her ability to communicate with you non-verbally will be efficient throughout this period. It's just a matter of you getting to know what her non-verbal communications mean.

She can communicate effectively with her body movements; she uses her head, legs, arms, hands and her facial expressions. These non-verbal communications are usually called 'baby cues'.

Non-verbal cues are small, moment-by-moment movements, which are not always easy to recognise or identify. Each cue is exactly the same as hearing one single word. Usually, you can't understand or get meaning from that unless you hear words put together in a sentence or from a gesture. So, just one non-verbal cue isn't enough to tell you what your baby's trying to communicate. For you to understand your baby, you need to watch all the non-verbal cues she's using in a given situation.

Let's look at a familiar scenario to learn how your baby might communicate. Many parents experience these types of playtime situations and their baby's behaviour can be confusing.

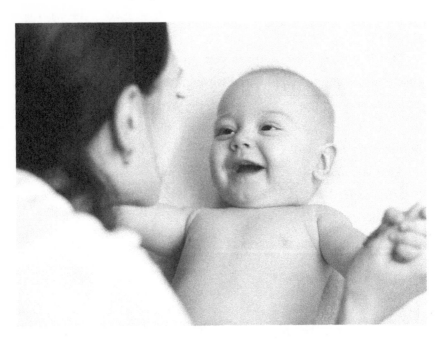

Scenario: confusing non-verbal cues

Your baby has just had her lunch and you decide she might like some playtime. You put her on her mat with some toys and plan to do a few quick chores while she plays. You look down at her and she lifts her face, gazes straight into your eyes and smiles. Her eyes are bright and shiny and she waves her arms towards you. She looks so sweet! She gives you a really strong message she wants you to play with her, so you decide the chores can wait.

You smile, touch and talk to each other for a few minutes. You show her some toys, but she's more interested in you than her toys. So, you sing a nursery rhyme using exciting facial expressions and finger actions. She really likes this game and for a minute or so she finds it very exciting, her eyebrows raise, she reaches out to you, smiles and joins in. You're both having so much fun.

Suddenly, and it seems for no reason, your baby starts to frown, she looks down and turns away. This confuses you because you were having such fun. You haven't got to the end of the rhyme and actions yet, so you keep going to cheer her along. She turns away even more. You follow her turned face and move in more closely to her and ask, 'What's wrong? Are you sad? Do you have a tummy ache?' Then you try to cheer her up by grasping her hands and trying to engage her in the nursery rhyme game again. You show her a happy face.

This time she pulls away from you, starts to flap her hands, shows you a sad face and cries.

What just happened? One minute you were having such fun together and now she doesn't want to play with you. Is she tired? Is she just fussy? Her behaviour seems so confusing.

Have you ever been in this situation? It's a common one, but even so it can be hard to interpret sometimes. So, here's what happened.

In the beginning of that time together, you can easily read her strong, non-verbal signals that she's ready to play.

Cues that your baby is ready to play

The cues are:

- raising her face to you
- gazing straight into your eyes
- reaching to you with her arms
- smiling
- her eyes are bright, shiny and alert.

These strong messages tell you she's ready to socialise. She's also alert and wide awake. That's the perfect time for her to play and socialise with you. You read her non-verbal language well. These types of baby cues are usually easy to read.

The next group of non-verbal messages she gives are not as easy to see and are often misinterpreted. When she starts to frown, look down and turn away, she's beginning to say, 'Wait a moment, this game is a bit too exciting.'

At this point in the game, she's not so bright and alert anymore. She's getting fretful, which gives you another clue that she's not ready for play or socialising at that moment. When she doesn't look at you with bright eyes, she's not ready to socialise or play.

Your baby can only take in little bits of stimulation at a time. Even though she enjoys the rhyme, finger play and your exciting facial expressions, every now and then she needs to take a break and relax from the game.

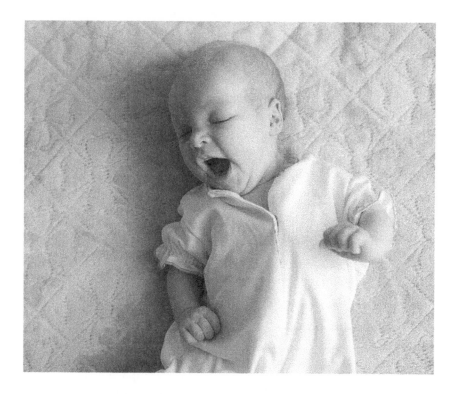

When she frowned, looked down and turned away, she was telling you, 'I need to stop for a moment.' Her behaviour is no different to your need to take a break when you've been working and concentrating hard. The only difference is that you verbally say, 'I need a break for a moment', and then you give yourself some time out.

When your baby gives these small, not so easy to see cues, it's time to sit back, give her some space and wait to see what happens next. When you can't see or you misinterpret her non-verbal cues, difficulties often occur in your communication with her.

It's easy to forget that your baby can't take in too much stimulation; to you, 1 or 2 minutes may not seem long at all, but it is for your baby. Her tolerance for the amount of stimulation she can cope with will vary, and your baby will let you know how much she can handle by giving you some non-verbal cues.

Your baby can only take in little bits of stimulation at a time.

Cues that your baby may be overstimulated

The cues are:

- frowning
- looking down
- looking away
- yawning
- putting her hand in her mouth
- touching her ear or head
- dull or glazed eyes.

In the example scenario we looked at, the difficulties started when her cues signalling her need for a rest were misinterpreted. It's natural to think your baby might be sad or have a tummy ache if she frowns or looks away. In fact, one of the first things parents are encouraged to think about when their baby cries or fusses is whether she has a tummy ache. Nothing could be further from the truth. Tummy aches don't cause every problem your baby has, but because there's a lot of talk between parents about stomach problems being the cause of unhappiness, it's often the first thing you think of. That's not your fault, but you can begin to think about things differently.

In this particular scenario, your baby was telling you that she needed some time out please. Naturally, when you misinterpret her behaviour as sadness or a possible tummy ache, you're going to want to cheer her up. So it's common to follow her turned head and move in close to her face, smile at her and try to continue the game in an effort to distract her.

Unfortunately, as soon as you do that she starts to give you some strong non-verbal messages, which may surprise you. Instead of cheering up, she indicates she has had enough.

Cues that your baby needs a break

The cues are:

- turning her head away from you
- starting to flap her hands
- arching her back
- showing you a very sad face
- crying.

These strong cues are hard to misinterpret. She's telling you, 'Stop trying to play with me.' It might be tempting to try harder still to cheer her up, but she can become even more upset.

So what happened? The same thing that happens to you when someone doesn't listen to you when you're overloaded and you need some peace and quiet for a moment – you are likely to get irritated or upset. Your baby is the same.

When she becomes overstimulated, your baby needs to take a break from playing. If her more subtle messages asking for some time out get misinterpreted, she'll send you some strong non-verbal cues saying, 'Stop playing! I'm even more stimulated and need you to soothe me now.' She's giving you clear messages that she needs your help.

When she gets to the point where she starts to cry, she's going to need your help to calm down. That means some soothing and reassurance to bring her back to a calm, relaxed state.

Here's what you do

When you're playing with her, it's nice to maintain both your own and her personal space. Personal space is usually about 20 to 30 centimetres from each other, except when you're being affectionate, kissing and hugging. This is especially important when she does need a break during your play or social time together.

When she gives you a non-verbal cue that means 'give me a moment', that's the time to sit back and wait until she gives you a non-verbal message that she's ready to socialise with you again. Tell her you're waiting in a quiet, soothing way.

When she's already overstimulated by the game you're playing, trying to continue may only stimulate her more. That's when she has to send you her strongest non-verbal cues.

Cues that your baby needs you to stop playing

The cues are:
- fussing
- crying
- flapping her arms
- arching away from you.

When she gives you these strong cues, she's saying, 'I need to stop the game now!'

Sometimes these types of cues are interpreted as having a tantrum or being naughty, and you might have been told she is bored and you try to do something even more exciting to distract her. But what your baby is really saying is, 'I'm overwhelmed and I need your help to calm down now.' The best way you can help her when she is distressed and upset is to use the soothing strategies outlined in Chapter 5: Why your baby cries.

Another snag that occurred in the example scenario is when you showed your baby a happy face and she showed you a sad face. When this happens, you become emotionally out of harmony. If it happens frequently, it can be confusing and uncomfortable for your baby.

She needs you to accept her sad feelings and then you can help her recover.

You do this by recognising she's sad, telling her she's sad, and then soothing and calming her to help her feel more in control of her emotions again. As she recovers, that's when you smile and tell her she's all right now and your harmony is restored.

Don't worry too much when your harmony gets disrupted, because it will happen quite often. No relationship is perfect and through incidents like this your baby learns that relationships have their ups and downs. You just need to figure out how to patch up the misinterpretation of her signals and move on.

One way you can do this is by learning your baby's non-verbal cues, how to communicate with each other and, when you get the message wrong, how to sort out the mix-up. The main message from this scenario is the importance of learning to interpret your baby's non-verbal cues.

When she's enjoying a game, enjoy it with her at her pace. Watch carefully for the first signs that she needs to have some time out. This is the signal for you to follow her lead and sit back and wait to see what she's going to do next.

There are a number of scenarios that could follow the break in the game you played:

- After she's had a chance to calm down she may want to play again.
- She may want to play a new game.
- She might be finished with playing completely and be ready for some quiet time before bed.

Watch carefully for the non-verbal messages that say, 'I want to play again and socialise.'

Cues your baby is ready for more play

The cues are:

- turning back to you
- bright eyes
- lifted eyebrows
- smiles
- arms stretched out.

Make sure to look for non-verbal messages that say, 'I'm done with playing.'

Cues your baby has had enough

The cues are:

- turning away from you
- dull face and eyes
- frown
- fussing.

Follow your baby's lead

The most important thing you can do is to follow your baby's lead. This actually makes understanding your baby easier because her non-verbal messages give you much more information about what she wants and needs.

Playing with her becomes easier as well, because you just go at her pace and enjoy watching what she enjoys. That's far more relaxing and fun for you than leading the game all the time. She'll tell you what she likes and, through this method of play, her brain will grow and develop even more effectively than if you provided a completely structured play routine. The bonus is that she's also learning that her communication is important because you are interested in what she's doing.

Watching her non-verbal cues will tell you when she wants you to join in and how she wants you to join in; you can relax and wait for her to tell you when she's finished. This type of communication between you will provide much more satisfying feeding and social times for both of you.

How your baby tells you when she's tired

You've probably already heard of 'tired signs'. Tired signs are another way of talking about non-verbal cues. But, like all non-verbal cues, you have to look at your baby's cues carefully because it's easy to misinterpret them if you don't put the cues together in the right way.

There's a bit more to interpreting tired signs than non-verbal cues, such as yawning, rubbing her eyes, pulling at her ears, making fists, kicking and fussing. Those cues can mean your baby just needs to take a short break from a social interaction, needs a position change, feed or cuddle. Remember the example scenario? There were lots of cues there that meant 'I just need a break', but those cues didn't necessarily mean 'I need a sleep', although they are often interpreted that way.

That's why it's important to think about tired signs as a collection of signs that include non-verbal cues.

You'll remember the information in the previous chapters about how sleep is controlled by the brain. The need for sleep builds up in her brain while your baby is awake. When she needs to go to sleep, her brain is going to tell her, 'It's time to go to sleep.' During sleep your baby has active sleep and quiet sleep – these are sleep states. Your baby's brain controls when she has each of these types of sleep. Her brain also controls when she naturally wakes up.

You can wake your baby out of sleep, of course, but you might notice that sometimes she's much harder to wake than at other times. That's because of the type of sleep she's in. She's much easier to wake in active sleep than when she's in quiet sleep.

During her awake times you'll notice that sometimes she's bright-eyed, alert and sociable; at other times she's alert and awake but fussy and wanting a feed, nappy change or just to be held. She's not very sociable during these wake periods. The final awake time is when she cries.

Just as her sleep states are controlled by her brain, so too are all of her wakeful states. These brain states are called 'states of consciousness' and they aren't under your control, although you can modify your baby's state by waking her up or soothing her when she cries.

As an adult, you have your own states of consciousness and your brain manages when you feel the need to sleep, your sleep cycles, when you naturally wake up, socialise and need to take a break from work and socialising. You can't control what your brain does when you're asleep – for example, you can't say, 'Hey, brain, I need to go from deep sleep to dream sleep now please' or 'Brain, I need to go from deep sleep to awake now please'. You need an alarm to do that. And, just like you, when your baby needs to go to sleep, her brain will move from an awake state into a drowsy state, getting her ready for sleep.

Think about yourself: you usually feel sleepy and drowsy before you go to sleep, don't you? You usually yawn, your eyes glaze over and if you looked in a mirror they would seem dull, your eyelids get heavy, your head might nod, and your body is fairly still. You may twitch and even jerk awake every now and then. These are those jerky movements and the tired signs that people say babies have.

Your baby is just the same and she also needs to feel drowsy before she goes to sleep. This means you are going to be thinking about and watching for several important things to determine when your baby is ready for sleep.

A tired sign formula

To make it easier to understand when to put your baby to bed, here's a special tired sign formula used by Tresillian:

Tresillian sleep formula
Brain state (state of consciousness)

+

Non-verbal cues

+

My baby's age and stage of sleep development

+

My baby's individuality

=

What my baby needs to go to sleep

Her individual needs

Your baby is an individual, so she has her own sleep needs. Hopefully, as you've been reading you've been getting a better idea of how sleep works and what her sleep needs are. It's essential to remember your baby will need different amounts of sleep as she grows, so that's an important clue to consider when you think about whether your baby is ready for sleep.

The first question to ask yourself is:

- 'How long ago was her last sleep?'

The following questions could be ones you ask yourself when your baby is about 6 weeks old to see if she is ready for sleep:

- What's her state of consciousness? Does she seem to:
  - be drowsy?
  - have heavy eyelids?
  - be getting quieter?
- Have you seen her giving you these types of non-verbal cues:
  - yawning?
  - heavy eyelids?
  - glazed or dull eyes?
  - sucking hands or putting her hands in her mouth?
  - still, quiet or not very alert?
  - fussy?
  - restless?

Take into account her age. When she's 6 weeks old, she will probably need a sleep 1 to 1½ hours after her last sleep.

Start to recognise your baby's individuality. Does your baby only stay awake an hour between feeds, or does she manage to stay awake and content for an hour and a half? You might be beginning to notice something special about her particular non-verbal cues when she's ready for bed.

When you use this type of tired sign formula, you can work out whether your baby is tired and ready for bed at each age and stage of her development. The more carefully you watch your baby, the better you will understand her individuality.

Each of your children will be different. When you are wondering when it's time to put your baby to bed, the non-verbal cues she gives will always go together with those other important clues in the tired sign formula to tell you what your baby needs.

Other non-verbal cue situations

Each situation you're in with your baby will be different. She will still give you the same types of non-verbal cues, but you have to look at them in relation to that particular situation. For example, she will give you lots of non-verbal cues during feeding times that can look like tired cues, but are they? During the play scenario, some of her non-verbal cues meant she wanted to play and others meant she needed a break from playing and socialising.

Cues during a feed
Some cues during both milk and solid feeds will invite you to:
- feed her
- stop feeding her
- socialise with her
- give her a break or rest
- slow down or speed up the feed
- help her to calm down.

Once again, the 'I need to have a break, please help me to calm down' cues can be misinterpreted as a tired sign or boredom during a feed. Usually, it can be that your baby just needs to have a rest or some space during the feed before having more to eat or finishing the feed because she's had enough to eat.

Non-verbal cues can mean many things during a feed, so it's important to watch your baby's non-verbal messages and wonder about what she's trying to tell you. Here are some common messages you could be getting through non-verbal cues.

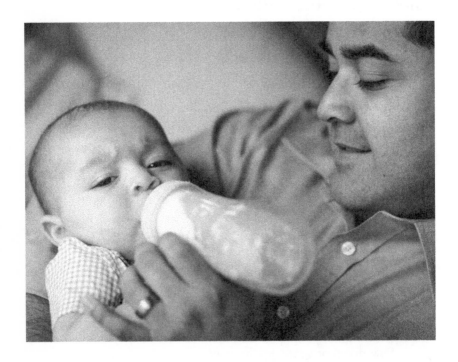

Understanding cues during a feed

- If she starts to cough or spit out the milk or solids, maybe the feed is going too fast for her.
- If she starts to smile and reach for you, she might need to stop the feed and have a social chat before she goes back and has a bit more to eat.
- If she starts to fuss, cry, pull away or push away, she might need to sit up or just have a cuddle.
- If it's a solid feed and she bangs her hand on the highchair table and reaches for the spoon, she's telling you she wants to hold the spoon on her own and try to feed herself. No matter how young she is, it's good to let her have a little try.
- If she hasn't finished her first mouthful before the next one is offered, she may arch her back, spit out her mouthful and push the spoon away. She's telling you she's not ready. Her mouth is too full. No one likes too much food in their mouth, it can make you gag. That can be frightening.

She's not being naughty when she does these things – she's just giving you clear non-verbal cues about her needs. From these examples you can see how easily non-verbal cues can be misinterpreted.

Once again, it's time to sit back, reassure her and wait for her to let you know if she wants some more to eat. Socialise with her if she needs that, try the spoon if she's ready to learn or end the meal if she's finished.

If you're confused about what your baby is trying to tell you, imagining what it's like to be in her situation can help you see it from her point of view. Here's another scenario where you are going to put yourself in your baby's shoes.

Scenario: misinterpreted cues during a feed

Imagine you can't speak any words yet and your parent is feeding you lunch. You like your lunch but you can't yet feed yourself, so you have no control over how fast the food is coming. It is coming a bit too fast, so you try to tell your parent with non-verbal cues that you need her to go slower and give you a break.

You give non-verbal cues to say, 'I need a breather', by:

- turning away
- banging on the highchair table
- putting your hand to your ear
- fussing
- frowning and kicking.

Unfortunately, your message is misinterpreted and your parent thinks you're full and have finished lunch. You reach for the food to try and tell her you're still hungry, but your parent misinterprets your non-verbal cues that meant you 'want a break' as tired signs. You cry for the food but, instead, you are picked up, rocked and told you are tired. Now you are really crying because you aren't drowsy or ready for sleep. Your parent is even more convinced you're tired because you're crying.

Your parent puts you to bed and tries some sleep and settling strategies to get you to sleep, but they don't work.

Your parent wonders if you have a sleep problem.

You are powerless to do anything.

This short scenario gives you another example of why you need to read non-verbal cues as they relate to the particular situation you are both in.

Right from birth your baby will give you lots of non-verbal cues about what she needs. When she's less than 3 months old and ready for a milk feed, she will usually show you all sorts of non-verbal cues together that mean she's hungry. She will:

- tuck her hands under her chin
- mouth and suck at her hands
- turn towards you if you touch her cheek (the rooting reflex)
- reach towards you
- curl her arms and legs up
- fuss or cry
- snuggle into your breast or body.

When she's full and had enough of her milk, she'll also show you a range of non-verbal cues:

- She'll be relaxed with straight arms and legs.
- Her hands won't be clenched.
- She may fall asleep.
- She may push or pull away from the breast or bottle.
- She may socialise to show you that the meal is over.

When she's older than 3 months, she will show you similar cues but she may add in stronger cues, such as:

- arching her back
- reaching or pointing to food when hungry
- the rooting reflex will disappear.

Non-verbal cues are your baby's powerful way of communicating with you. Once you watch her carefully, learn how to read her non-verbal language and understand how she's communicating with you, you'll both enjoy a much more satisfying relationship.

Anya's story (mother of Otis, 2)

My son was 4 months old when I went to Tresillian – and I wish I'd gone sooner. I was incredibly sleep-deprived and almost at rock bottom. I'd suffered severe morning sickness throughout my pregnancy. I wasn't able to keep anything down and even had to go to hospital several times for cannulas to stop me dehydrating.

By the time I delivered Otis, I was completely depleted and was suddenly at home by myself with a crying baby to care for. My husband works long hours and travels a lot and my family live interstate, so I felt incredibly alone. I was trying to breastfeed him but he woke so regularly for feeds that it seemed like he wasn't getting enough milk. I tried sleep consultants and my GP but the one-size-fits-all approach just didn't fit me at all.

Once I got to Tresillian, it was like I could take a big breath of fresh air and allow the experts to help me. The nurses were so empathetic; they looked at every aspect of my situation and worked with me to find a solution. I also consulted with a psychologist and a psychiatrist, as I was suffering a lot of anxiety.

I was finding it hard to settle him, so the nurses helped me understand his tired signs. I realised I was completely missing them. Otis would get really overactive and seemed to run at double speed when he was starting to get tired. I was taking that as a sign he wanted more play, but it was completely the opposite!

As he was only 4 months, the nurses advised arm settling, which I was really relieved about. I didn't want to put him down crying and leave him to settle himself as it just didn't sit right with me. I would rock him until he was really drowsy then put him in his cot and sit with him until he fell asleep. When he cried, I would pick him up and start the process again. I felt like such an awesome mum when he fell asleep happy, warm and comforted.

Otis is now 2 and is sleeping perfectly. It took me until he was 1 to really recover from my pregnancy, but now I feel fine and am really enjoying being a mum. In our situation there was nothing really wrong with Otis – it was all me, and my first-time mum anxieties, coupled with severe exhaustion.

Key message

- Your baby gives many small, moment-by-moment non-verbal cues, but a single cue is not always easy to recognise or identify as a message of what she needs. You have to put her non-verbal cues together, just like stringing words together to form a sentence.

- Your baby won't be able to communicate her needs to you with words until well into her second year, and even then she will have some trouble telling you how she feels and what she needs. Your baby can't cope with large amounts of stimulation, and this will vary according to her age and her temperament. Trust your baby and as you get to know her, she will let you know how much stimulation she can handle.

- Watch your baby's non-verbal cues during a feed and consider what she's trying to tell you. Non-verbal cues can mean many things during a feed, so when you watch, understand and respond to her in the right way, you'll both enjoy meal times much more.

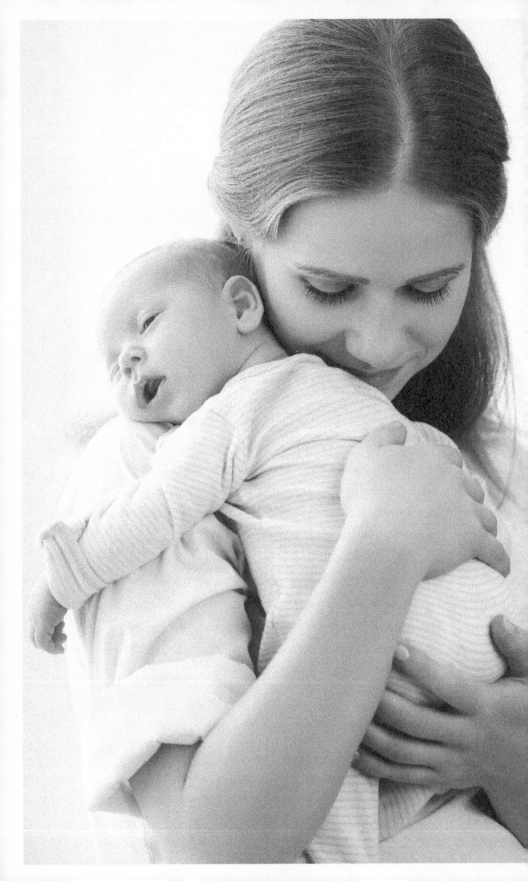

CHAPTER 7

Working on sleep problems: Birth to 6 months

So far, we've looked at your baby's normal sleep development, normal crying and how your baby communicates through non-verbal cues. It's good to know what's normal because it helps you decide whether or not you and your baby have any problems with sleep and settling.

You may have decided that your baby and you are perfectly normal and feel relieved to know that by setting up a routine and following along with your baby's normal sleep development, everything will be fine. But if you've got to this point and decided that things aren't quite right or your sleep routines may not be working in the way you thought they would, it's time to figure out how to adjust the parts of sleep that aren't working for you and your baby.

In this chapter, we will use Tresillian's sleep and settling strategies as a guideline, with options to help you manage your baby's sleep. Note that Tresillian does not recommend or use controlled crying for babies of any age.

Tresillian does not recommend or use controlled crying for babies of any age.

Birth to 3 months

As you know, for the first three months your baby's sleep rhythms are still maturing, so she will sometimes require some gentle help settling to sleep and soothing back to sleep when she wakes between sleep cycles. This is perfectly normal during these early months.

It might be tempting to think that your baby has a sleeping problem during these first three months because she needs some help to relax off to sleep and keeps waking so frequently, but usually, it's all part of your baby's normal sleep development.

In the first month after birth, your baby will have a semi-regular, 2- to 4-hourly routine, around the 24-hour clock. Through the first month, 95 per cent of babies cry when they wake during a sleep and need a calm and gentle response before they can resettle and return to sleep.

From birth to 3 months, you are helping your baby establish her day–night rhythms and beginning to put in place a flexible feeding, socialising and sleep routine (see Chapter 1: How sleep works). During these months, bedtime routines, settling to sleep and resettling strategies will be simple and responsive to her needs.

Your baby may be quite sleepy for the first week or two after birth but, of course, she has her own personality and you may discover that she has quite different ideas! Some babies can be more wakeful than others, but this doesn't mean there's something wrong. These are just individual differences. You are finding out who she is and what she likes and doesn't like. You are getting to know each other and that takes a little bit of time.

What your baby needs most at this stage is lots of cuddling, frequent feeds and a quick, soothing and sensitive response to her cries and distress.

People often say you will spoil your baby if you do that, but it's not true. Once again, these beliefs emerged from the early-20th century 'childcare experts' who promoted the idea that babies should be pushed into independence from birth, and that responding to crying made a child whiney and spoilt.

The opposite is true: the more love and sensitive attention you provide your baby when she is distressed, the better she will be able to cope with distress later on.

Throughout the first month, focus on these aspects of caring for your new baby:

- Adjust to your new life with your baby.
- Begin to get to know your baby.
- Hold her close to you, especially when she's distressed.
- Feed her when she's hungry – this can be every 2 to 5 hours.
- Watch her carefully and get to know her non-verbal cues (see Chapter 6: How your baby communicates).
- Socialise and play with her when she is in a quiet, alert state (see Chapter 6: How your baby communicates).
- Settle her into her bed to sleep and gently and calmly help her back to sleep when she wakes after a sleep cycle.

By 3 weeks old, your baby will start to cry more as she moves into her normal developmental crying phase (see Chapter 5: Why your baby cries) and this may disrupt her sleep at some periods of the day, usually in the late afternoon or evening.

Routines. Once your baby is 2 to 3 months of age, her day–night rhythms have established and she's more awake and sociable. You can probably begin to develop a more predictable yet flexible rhythm to your day during this time.

Your day will usually be organised around feeding, socialising and sleeping. A flexible rhythm may look something like this.

From birth to 3 months, help your baby establish her day–night rhythms and begin to put in place flexible routines.

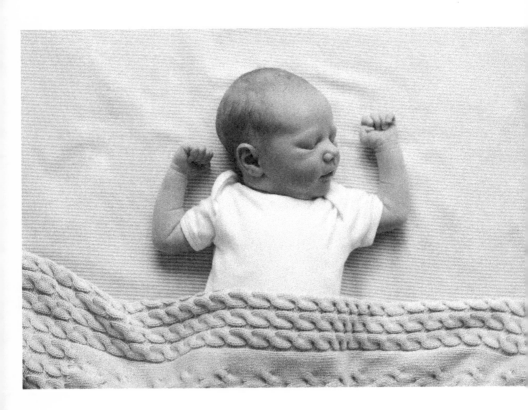

Scenario: a flexible feeding and sleeping routine

Your baby wakes after a sleep of about 3½ hours. She shows you by her non-verbal cues that she's hungry (see Chapter 6: How your baby communicates). You breastfeed her or give her a formula feed.

During the feed she falls asleep, so you decide to change her nappy and she wakes up again. She shows you by her non-verbal cues that she's still hungry, so you give her some more milk. Finally, she shows you she's full, alert and happy.

After her feed, her eyes are bright and shiny, she's smiling at you and her arms are reaching for you. She's ready to play and socialise. You both enjoy talking to each other for a few minutes before she starts to look away. You sit back and wait to see if she wants to talk and play again. She wants to keep socialising and this back-and-forth play and time out cycle continues for another 10 minutes. Finally, she becomes very fussy and she's finished socialising.

You can see she looks drowsy. You check your watch and note she's been awake for 1 hour and 15 minutes. You know she usually doesn't last much longer than that. She's showing non-verbal tired cues. You decide it's time for bed.

You use responsive settling strategies to put her to sleep and when she wakes during her sleep, you use the same strategies to resettle her. This time she sleeps for 1½ hours and wakes up hungry. You can't resettle her, so you feed her and she falls asleep again. You settle her and she returns to sleep.

You repeat this flexible rhythm throughout the day. At night, you don't play or socialise with her.

In this scenario, you were able to wake your baby during the feed and she took some more milk from you because she was still hungry. If she falls asleep during a feed, it's important to consider whether your baby might be hungry and want some more milk. Remember, though, that during these first few months your baby will often fall asleep immediately after a feed and this is quite normal.

It's perfectly okay to leave her asleep if she falls asleep during the feed, and perhaps feed her more frequently if she wakes and seems hungry. You will have to look for her cues that tell you when she's hungry.

The predictable thing about this flexible rhythm is that you:

- use the same settling strategies
- keep feed times in a flexible rhythm guided by her hunger cues
- use the same soothing strategies when she's distressed (see Chapter 5: Why your baby cries)
- follow her cues (see Chapter 6: How your baby communicates)
- try to place her in the same place to sleep
- change her nappy before, in the middle or at the end of her feed
- have her bath time around the same time each day.

During these first three months, your baby may occasionally manage to soothe herself to sleep. You can try wrapping her firmly in a cotton wrap and putting her in her crib in a drowsy state, but she may still wake after a sleep cycle and require resettling.

Settling your baby in the early months

Settling your baby in the first three months isn't complicated. She needs you to be patient while she matures and develops her normal sleep rhythms and cycles. This requires a sensitive and responsive approach to help her structure her day so that it's calm, predictable and sociable, as well as gentle, soothing approaches to help her go to sleep and settle.

Remember that Tresillian doesn't use controlled crying. Instead, the focus is on responding sensitively to your baby.

Young babies shouldn't be left to cry inconsolably on their own. Crying is a call for comfort and help. A young baby will not 'learn to sleep' by being left to cry. A baby will just experience more distress if she doesn't get the support and response she needs.

Once again, put yourself in your baby's shoes. If you cry in bed prior to sleep, how do you feel? No one likes crying themselves to sleep, that's exhausting and miserable.

If you try to put your baby to bed awake and she's unable to settle on her own, leaving her to cry as a settling strategy is highly stressful for you both. The evidence suggests that she will just learn to stop crying rather than learn to sleep.

The strategies recommended by Tresillian encourage you to respond promptly and sensitively to your baby's distress, her non-verbal cues and her states of consciousness, which are:

- wakefulness
- drowsiness
- active and quiet sleep.

Tresillian follows Red Nose recommendations on safe sleeping for your baby to reduce the risk of Sudden Unexpected Deaths in Infancy (SUDI), including SIDS.

Safe sleeping guidelines

- Sleep baby on the back from birth, not on tummy or side.
- Sleep baby with head and face uncovered.
- Keep baby smoke-free before birth and after.
- Provide a safe sleeping environment, night and day.
- Sleep baby in their own safe sleeping place in the same room as an adult caregiver for the first 6 to 12 months.
- Breastfeed baby.

Responsive Settling techniques

Tresillian uses a method to settle your baby called 'Responsive Settling'. The following variously named techniques are suitable for your baby through each stage of her development: use the gentle soothing-in-arms technique for birth to 3 months; and then the hands-on settling technique (see page 153) for when your baby has established a predictable day–night routine, at around 3 to 6 months. (See Chapter 8 for information about Responsive Settling techniques for babies older than 6 months.)

Remember, Tresillian does not use controlled crying.

Responsive Settling: soothing-in-arms technique

Use the soothing-in-arms technique for the early weeks of your baby's life, when she's developing her day–night rhythms and doesn't always have the ability to self-settle to sleep or back to sleep when she wakes. This is a gentle technique you can use from birth to 3 months, especially if you have a very unsettled baby.

Soothing-in-arms technique

1. Hold your baby in your arms until she falls asleep or becomes drowsy.
2. Use gentle, rhythmic patting, rocking, stroking, talking or soft singing before putting your baby into her cot when she is asleep or drowsy. These repetitions of soothing sounds and actions are comforting and signal relaxation and sleep.
3. If your baby wakes after a sleep cycle, you may need to re-settle her using any of the strategies listed in step 2.

These strategies help your baby settle and calm to sleep when she's having trouble sleeping. These early months are the time when she needs the most help and reassurance from you.

By 3 months of age, your baby will probably have progressed through the normal developmental crying stage and her crying is reduced to about 1 hour per day. Her sleep rhythms will have matured and she will be shifting into a new phase of development.

These early months are the time
when she needs the most help
and reassurance from you.

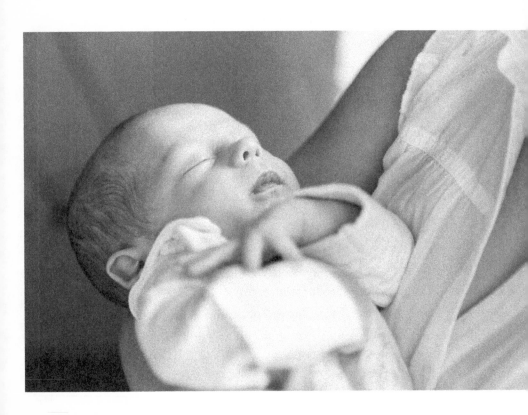

3 to 6 months

At 3 months of age, your baby has a major developmental growth spurt. Her body is much more under her own control and her little hands are becoming useful at last. She enjoys looking at her hands and will start to use them.

You will notice she spends more time awake and she is much more sociable and interested in interacting with you. She loves to gaze at you.

If you watch her carefully, she will gaze at you, move her body and vocalise almost in time with you when you gaze at her, speak, smile and play. While she's doing this with you, she's developing her thinking skills, and her social and emotional development is evolving.

At about 4 months, she'll begin to shift her gaze from you and look at toys when you show them to her. She will become more interested in toys as she moves towards 6 months.

Her wakeful periods will last from 1½ hours to as long as 2½ hours, and her daytime naps will be approximately 2 hours long. These lengths

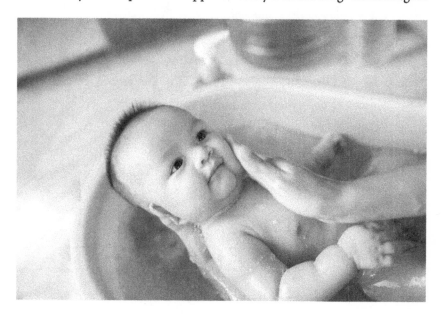

of time are averages only and they will match her age and development. For example, your 3-month-old baby will have longer and more frequent naps than a 6-month-old baby, and she will have shorter wakeful periods than a 6-month-old baby.

Daily routine

Once your baby gets to 3 months she is more awake and alert, so her routines begin to have a more predictable pattern. But her routines remain flexible and you need to adapt them to her age and development.

Sample routine for your 3-month-old baby

- Wake at 5 am, have an early milk feed and start the day, or return to sleep
- Have a milk feed every 3 to 4 hours
- Play and socialise with you after a milk feed
- Perhaps have some floor play on her own or sit watching you while you do something
- Go for a walk in the pram or visit friends
- Carefully watch your baby for when she gets drowsy and use your tired sign formula (see page 125). Remember, it's best to put her to bed when she's in a drowsy state.
- Have a 2-hour sleep
- Have a bath and her bedtime routine in the evening and settle for the night
- One to two milk feeds overnight, usually at about 10 pm or 11 pm and another at 1 am or 2 am.

By 6 months of age, her meals and bedtime routines will be beginning to look a little like the rest of the family's. Your 4- to 6-month-old baby's routine may look like this:

Sample routine for your 4- to 6-month-old baby

- Wake at 5 am and start the day after her early morning milk feed, or maybe return to sleep
- Morning tea milk feed (at 6 months, you may have started her on solids)
- Playtime includes social time with you enjoying toys together, singing songs, reading books, floor play on her own or sitting in her highchair watching you while you prepare your lunch and do some chores
- Go for a walk in the pram, visit friends, baby playgroup
- Carefully watch your baby for when she gets drowsy and use your tired sign formula (see page 125). Remember, it's best to put her to bed when she's in a drowsy state.
- Lunch milk feed (at 6 months, you may have started her on solid food)
- Have a 2-hour sleep twice a day
- Afternoon milk feed
- Have a bath and her bedtime routine in the evening and settle for the night
- Evening milk feed
- She may still want a milk feed overnight, usually at about 10 pm to 11 pm or at about 1 am to 2 am.

Disruptions. Routines don't always go smoothly and are easily disrupted by changes in the family environment, illness and going on holidays (see Chapter 4: Creating a conducive sleep environment). Disruptions also occur to your routine when you have busy days out and about. For example, shopping centres are highly stimulating with lots of people, noise and bright lights.

It's hard for your baby to sleep under such circumstances. Again, put yourself in your baby's position and imagine what it would be like to try and sleep in a busy shopping centre when your sleep is still developing. Too much stimulation will disrupt her routine. Small amounts are fine.

Sleep difficulties. It's thought that about 60 to 70 per cent of 4-month-old babies will be able to sleep continuously for episodes of about 5 hours a night on most nights of the week and wake two to three times during these episodes (see Chapter 2: Sleeping longer through the night). These babies are able to settle themselves back to sleep after an awakening, but about 30 per cent of babies cry out when they wake.

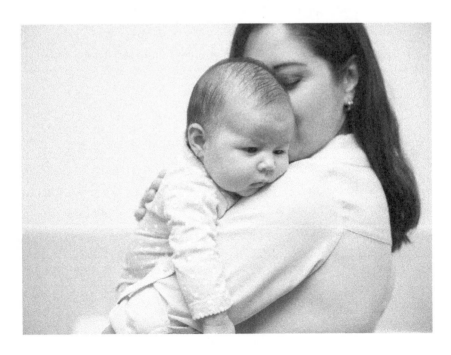

It's during this period of your baby's life that you and she may find yourselves falling into some sleep habits that may contribute to sleep difficulties later on. The real issue about sleep difficulties is not that your baby wakes up at night or during her daytime naps, because that's normal, but working out why she calls out when she wakes. The ability to stop calling to you when she wakes is believed to be a normal sleep maturational process that will develop over time.

By 3 to 4 months, about 70 per cent of babies will have reduced the number of times they call out to about once per night, on most nights of the week. If your baby keeps calling out to you many more times than this, it's because she's still developing the capacity to settle on her own. She may still need some gentle and responsive help from you.

There are two types of well-recognised sleep problems that occur over the next few months. The first is that your baby has difficulties going to bed and falling asleep on her own. And the second is your baby can't return to sleep on her own after waking between sleep cycles.

There are lots of different reasons why sleep problems occur, but one thing is for sure: it's always a combination of reasons that involve both you and your baby (see Chapter 3: The two sides of your sleep problems).

After your baby is about 3 months old, one of the most important things you can do is to help her start to soothe herself to sleep at the beginning of each sleep.

Going to bed awake

Once the first three months have passed and your baby has settled into a more regular day–night rhythm, she is developing a greater capacity to soothe herself to sleep at bedtime and when she wakes during the night and her naps. You can support her sleep development by using some simple settling strategies.

Calming bedtime routine

- Carefully watch for when your baby gets drowsy and use your tired sign formula (see page 125). Remember, it's best to put her to bed when she's drowsy.
- Wrap her firmly but comfortably in a cotton wrap, with her arms flexed against her chest so she can get her hands to her mouth in case she wants to suck them. This will help her to soothe herself. Leave enough room in her wrap for her to move her legs. You don't want to wrap her tightly like an Egyptian mummy. You can imagine it would be an unnatural and uncomfortable way to sleep, with your arms pinned straight down your sides.
- Speak to her in a calm, soothing and low voice while you're getting her ready for bed and putting her into her crib. Sing a lullaby if you enjoy singing.
- Put her to bed in the same familiar place.
- If it's daytime, you don't need to make the room totally dark. A little daylight is fine.
- If it's night-time, ensure the light in the room isn't stimulating, such as light from the TV, computers, smartphones or tablets (see Chapter 1: How sleep works).
- Give her a reassuring kiss or stroke her head and leave her to see if she can settle.

Firstly, to address any potential future difficulties with her going to bed, you can start by putting your baby to bed awake. This is a good time to begin with a simple, soothing and calm bedtime routine.

While she is trying to settle herself, she will make lots of little noises, like grunts and snorts, sometimes a louder squeak. It's okay to leave her alone while she does that, as she is probably transitioning from a drowsy state to another sleep state (see Chapter 2).

It's important not to interrupt her during that process. So, unless she starts to fuss and cry loudly, just leave her alone to give her the opportunity to go to sleep by herself. If you can manage to hold back and allow her to have a good try, this will help her to start to develop a really good sleep routine.

For example, if you take a peep at her as she moves from a drowsy state to an active sleep state, she may still seem awake to you because her eyelids may be fluttering, her breathing may be irregular and she may be moving and twitching. It's best to leave her alone at this stage so she can move from active sleep into a quiet, deeper sleep state.

If your baby doesn't manage to fall asleep on her own when you put her to bed awake, this may be because she is still developmentally immature. The capacity to settle on her own to sleep and during sleep develops over time, and each baby is different. Even so, from around the third month of your baby's life it's worthwhile to give her the opportunity to go to bed awake and settle on her own.

Waking between sleep cycles

The second sleep problem that may occur over the next few months is that your baby may find soothing herself back to sleep after waking between sleep cycles quite difficult.

Once your baby is 3 to 6 months old and she is developing the ability to soothe herself to sleep, she also has the ability to sleep for 2 to 3 hours at a stretch during the day and 5 hours at night. During these prolonged stretches, she may manage to soothe herself back to sleep between sleep cycles at least once. When you put her to bed awake and give her the opportunity to soothe herself to sleep, this may help her to soothe herself when she wakes between sleep cycles. But even at this young age, your baby won't be able to do this at every sleep; or she may not be able to do it at all.

There is some debate about why some babies aren't able to soothe themselves to sleep. These are the two possible reasons:

1. Some babies' sleep development is more immature than other babies'. They need more help to fall asleep and also to go back to sleep when they wake between sleep cycles.
2. Other babies' sleep development may be maturing normally, but their parents might not be giving them the space they need to practice settling themselves to sleep. Some parents respond too quickly when their baby wakes during the night.

Both these reasons are very common, and neither you nor your baby is to blame. This is a bit like the chicken or the egg scenario.

If your baby's sleep development is a little immature, then of course you're going to attend to her and try to put her to sleep. What can then happen is your baby can begin to associate your presence and your method of putting her to sleep with going to sleep.

Or you might mistake the little noises she makes when she wakes as calls for help, and you go to her too quickly. Once again, she begins to associate needing you to be with her in order for her to go back to sleep.

These are called 'sleep associations', which basically means that whatever you do to put your baby to sleep – such as feed her or hold her until she's asleep and then put her into her bed when she's asleep – she will expect the same from you each time she wakes up, even throughout the night.

The best way to manage sleep at this age is to continue with the same calm, soothing and responsive strategies you used during the first three months but add in a little more structure to help her settle.

Responsive Settling: hands-on settling technique

Once your baby has established a predictable day–night rhythm and you can see she has a beginning capacity to self-settle, from between 3 to 6 months, start incorporating the hands-on settling technique in your routine.

Wrap your baby with her arms up on her chest so she can move them to her mouth if she needs to; or use a sleeping bag with fitted armholes, and no hood (following Red Nose safe baby sleeping bag guidelines).

Hands-on settling technique

1. Talk quietly and cuddle your baby to help her calm.
2. Place your baby in her bed when she is in a calm and drowsy state but still awake.
3. Comfort your baby with gentle 'shhh' sounds and gentle rhythmic patting, rocking or stroking until she is calm or asleep.
4. If your baby becomes or stays distressed, pick her up for a cuddle until she's calm or asleep before putting her back in her bed.
5. Stay with your baby until she is asleep.

During her first six months, your baby is developing rapidly in all areas: physically, emotionally, mentally and socially. Just like walking and talking, sleep is one of those areas of development that matures over time. You wouldn't expect your baby to begin walking or talking to you at 3 months, and sleep is just the same. It takes quite a long time

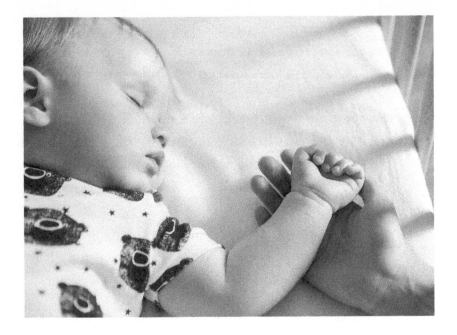

before your baby will sleep through the night, and just like walking and talking, it takes some baby's longer than others to develop the capacity to sleep longer and self-settle. Some parents like guidelines to support their baby's sleep development, especially when sleep seems to be a problem for both them and their baby.

As this chapter outlined, there is quite a steady development in your baby's ability to settle to sleep and self-settle back to sleep during the first six months. She starts off after birth with very little capacity to settle herself and needs lots of help. By 3 months of age, she's beginning to put herself to sleep and settle herself during the night, and that's when you might start to get some longer sleeps. With your loving help and support, and using the Tresillian Responsive Settling techniques, by 6 months she may be able to go to bed and fall asleep, then self-settle on her own during the night (see Chapter 2: Sleeping longer through the night for length of sleep times).

Jillian's story (mother of Luca, 11 months)

If I'm honest, the sleep issues with my son were mainly to do with my husband and me. My son would wake after 40 minutes during the day and every 2 hours at night. During the day, I would just assume that he'd had enough sleep after 40 minutes and would get him up.

As time went on, he was crying more and more and sleeping even less. I was completely exhausted and when Luca was around 4 months old, I realised I needed to get help. I spoke to my GP and booked a Day Stay at Tresillian.

My husband and I are against controlled crying – we wanted to ensure we weren't abandoning him, so we responded to his every cry. What we didn't realise was that often babies need to make noises to go to sleep. We were actually overdoing trying to settle him for every sleep and were disturbing his ability to learn how to settle himself.

At Tresillian, the nurse sat with us while our son tried to self-settle. She helped us distinguish his noises and showed us which ones were him just settling himself and which ones were actual distress and required our input.

For the first nap, we sat outside the door for a few minutes while he grizzled (although it felt like years). After 5 minutes, he really started to get upset, so she told us to go in and comfort him. She said, 'Don't pick him up. Be calm, go in slowly, put your hand on him and shush/pat him. If he's unwrapped, then wrap him back up, but don't make a big production out of it.'

So, we did all that and waited until he was calm, then we went out again. We had to keep going in and out for about half an hour but eventually, he went to sleep.

'And that's how you do it,' the nurse said. It was a definite eye-opener.

When we got home, we kept practising and after a few weeks he worked it out and he started settling himself to sleep. I also had to help resettle him between naps as he would wake after 40 minutes but, after a while, he learned how to transition between sleep cycles and I wouldn't hear a peep. The first day he did a 90-minute nap, I didn't know myself!

These days, he's doing two good naps a day and even though he still wakes every so often overnight, we're all getting reasonable sleep. Although it was hard to hear, I'm glad that I found out early that I wasn't doing it right and how to fix it.

Key message

- For the first three months, your baby's sleep rhythms are still maturing, so she will sometimes require some gentle help settling to sleep and soothing back to sleep when she wakes between sleep cycles.
- At 3 months of age, your baby is much more sociable and loves to interact with you. She is much more awake and alert during the day and her feeding, socialising and sleeping routines begin to have a more predictable pattern. At this age, she may stay awake for 1 to 2 hours at a time and have 2-hour naps.
- Between 3 and 6 months, your baby will develop a predictable day–night rhythm and have the beginning capacity to self-settle.
- By the time your baby reaches 6 months, her awake periods will be longer, but she will still have two to three naps of varying lengths during the day. At 6 months, many babies have the ability to sleep for a 6-hour stretch at least once at night. Your baby may have started solids and have a solid breakfast with you in the morning, she may have lunch, snacks and dinner, and she will have an evening bedtime with a routine.

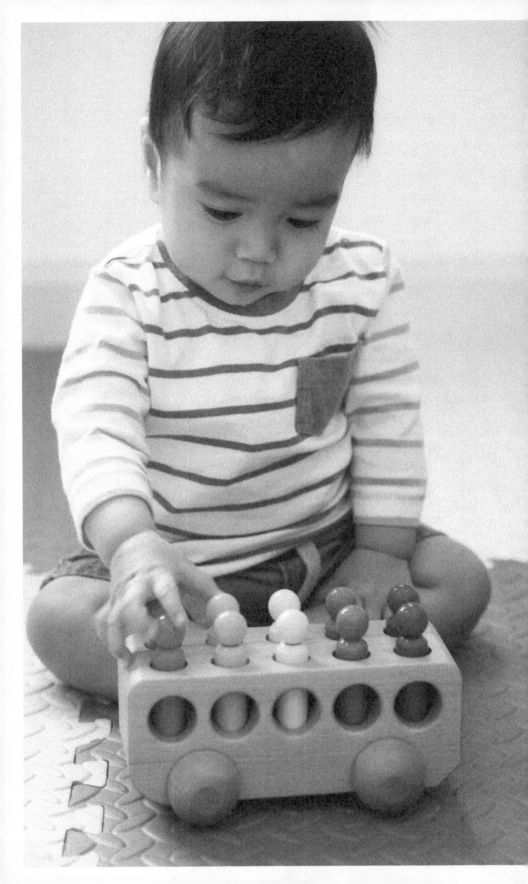

CHAPTER 8

Working on sleep problems: 6 to 12 months

So your baby has reached the second half of her first year. During these six months, she will be much more alert to her surroundings.

You will start her on some solid food and this is the exciting time when she begins to get mobile all on her own. It's time to start thinking about moving your precious bits and pieces out of her way because she's curious, and the closer she gets to 9 months and the better her mobility becomes, the more she will want to explore her surroundings.

She will want to look at and touch everything! At this age, she is so inquisitive and will follow your every movement. She loves to look at leaves and trees, at the toys you show her and at her older brothers and sisters.

She will still want to put everything in her mouth because her hands don't quite do their job yet. And some babies will continue to mouth toys right up to the age of 12 months.

Your baby shows enormous enjoyment and delight in your company and doesn't like to be left alone at all, and you can't blame her for that. She's fallen totally in love with you. You are her favourite person in the world and when you're not with her, she feels sad and misses you. She really does need to keep her eye on you, so once she's able to crawl, she'll follow you as fast as she can.

This attachment to you is a completely normal part of her development. Over the previous six months, you've both built a close and loving relationship. For your baby, it's the first time she's ever experienced falling in love with someone. Now she wants to stay close and do whatever you're doing, including following you to the toilet, as annoying as that is. It can also sometimes mean not leaving you to go to sleep!

During this second six months, your baby's sleep patterns usually change very little. She will continue to sleep continuously for stretches of about 5 to 6 hours a night on most nights and wake two to three times (see Chapter 2: Sleeping longer through the night). She may be able to settle herself back to sleep after waking. By 12 months of age, your baby may be able to sleep for two 6-hour periods during the night. She will still wake one to three times and hopefully resettle herself without your help.

However, there are some major developmental stages during these six months that can disrupt your baby's sleep, even if she's slept well up to this point. Namely, these are crawling and separation anxiety.

In this chapter, we look at routines for 6- to 12-month-old babies and strategies to help your baby settle if she has problems going to sleep or self-settling when she wakes after a sleep cycle.

6 to 9 months

By now, your baby's day will be moving into a more comfortable pattern. You will both work around feeding, socialising and sleeps, but your baby will be ready for some solid food and will begin to have breakfast, lunch and dinner with her milk feed. She's moving slowly towards fitting in with the family's mealtime schedules.

She will have two sleeps a day as she is much more alert and awake. Her night-time sleep periods will stretch for about 10 to 12 hours, with one prolonged sleep of about 6 hours.

At 6 months of age, she will be more interested in toys and she will enjoy looking at toys when you show them to her. She still won't play a game with you and the toy – she will look at the toy carefully, hold and investigate it, then put it in her mouth. She may seem totally oblivious to you while she has the toy.

At this age, she still likes action songs and a little rough-and-tumble play with you. She gets to know action songs now and will anticipate the actions of the song or nursery rhyme and laugh when she knows something exciting is about to happen. As you can see your facial expressions, voice, touch and emotions are a vital source of her social, emotional and intellectual development. This is what she enjoys most for play and social time. As she reaches 9 months, she will shift her attention to playing with you and the toys.

Daily routine

Any routine you develop for your baby needs to suit your family, your cultural background and your lifestyle. Most importantly, your baby's day needs to have a predictable yet flexible pattern that keeps her comfortable and secure and maintains her sleep–wake rhythms.

Between 6 and 9 months, your baby's meals and bedtime routines will begin to look more like the rest of the family's.

Sample routine for your 6- to 9-month-old baby

- Your baby may still wake as early as 5 am (or around sunrise) and have an early milk feed. She may start the day then or return to sleep for a little while. This depends on the type of person your baby is. Unfortunately, she may not share your enjoyment of a sleep-in.
- Breakfast solids and a milk feed. This is the age when she likes to start holding her bottle and spoon, patting your breast. She wants to take a more active part in feeding.
- Playtime includes social time with you, enjoying and handling colourful toys that make sounds and vary in texture, singing songs with actions, crawling about or sitting in her highchair watching you while you do some work. She'll enjoy a chat while she chews a toy.
- Going for a walk in her pram, visiting friends, baby playgroup
- Morning tea (perhaps fruit) and a drink of water
- Carefully watch your baby for when she gets drowsy and use your tired sign formula (see page 125). Remember, it's best to put her to bed when she's in a drowsy state.
- A nap of about 2 to 2½ hours
- Lunch solids and a milk feed
- Another playtime
- Carefully watch your baby for when she gets drowsy and use your tired sign formula (see page 125). Remember, it's best to put her to bed when she's in a drowsy state.
- A nap of about 1 to 2 hours
- Afternoon tea (perhaps fruit) and a drink of water
- Playtime

- On some days, if she's very tired, your baby made need a shorter third nap.
- Dinner solids and a milk feed
- Quiet, wind-down cuddle time
- A bath and her bedtime routine in the evening and settle for the night
- She may still want one milk feed overnight.

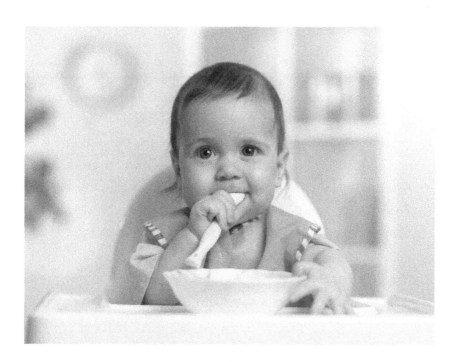

9 to 12 months

Your baby is really blossoming. She knows her name and turns to you when you call. If you've established a familiar and flexible routine, she will generally find most days predictable. And this will help her sleep at night.

Your day is still centred on feeding, socialising and sleeps, but more and more she's fitting into family schedules, which makes organising your day a little easier.

The variety of food she's eating is much more interesting, plus she can begin to feed herself with finger foods and she enjoys holding the spoon. If she manages to put the spoon near the food she'll make a mess, but how can she learn to use a spoon without making mistakes and a mess at the same time?

She will start by aiming at the bowl and dipping the spoon into the food, and by 12 months she may even get some food into her mouth. While she's doing this, she's learning so much about holding the spoon in her hand just the right way, how to move her arms, and coordinating when to open her mouth at just the right time. It's hard to get the spoon into the bowl and then into her mouth. There's so much she has to learn to coordinate. That takes a lot of practice to get right. She will also love reaching out to grab food and feel very clever when she picks it up and puts it in her mouth.

Her sleep remains pretty much the same, with two daytime naps. Her night-time sleep periods now have the potential to last anywhere from 6 to 8 hours at one stretch, with another short sleep. She will still have one to three brief awakenings and will hopefully resettle herself.

She is much more mobile, and if you haven't moved all your precious belongings out of her reach, now is the time to do so. You need to keep her safe, as she has no idea about danger. During this period, her memory is short and she doesn't have the intellectual ability to remember or understand verbal rules, such as 'No, don't touch that'.

She's inquisitive and will want to inspect everything. When she keeps going back to an electric power point or to touch something you've left within her reach that you don't want her to touch, she's not being naughty; she's being normal. It's best to make your house safe so you don't have to spend your time distressed and worried that she's getting into things she shouldn't be touching.

A good website for information on how to keep your baby safe at home is Kidsafe (kidsafensw.org/).

At 9 to 12 months, your baby's intellectual, social and emotional development is flourishing. Playing is the business of childhood and your baby is really busy now. Instead of just being totally absorbed in a toy when you give her one, she shares your attention with the toys. This means she shows you toys, shares the toy with you and will play with you for a few minutes at most. Remember, she doesn't have a long attention span.

Some of the interesting things she enjoys doing from 9 months onwards include:

- pulling toys with a string
- playing peek-a-boo
- clapping hands
- stacking toys
- listening to songs and music
- playing pat-a-cake.

If you hide a toy under a cover while she's watching, she may be able to find it straight away. This is a major development!

She also loves letting go of and dropping toys – especially from her highchair. People often think your baby is being naughty when she does this, but she's learning a new skill. She's learning to open her little hand and let go of something. Why not have some fun while she's doing it? She's learning about gravity at the same time. And yes, it does get a

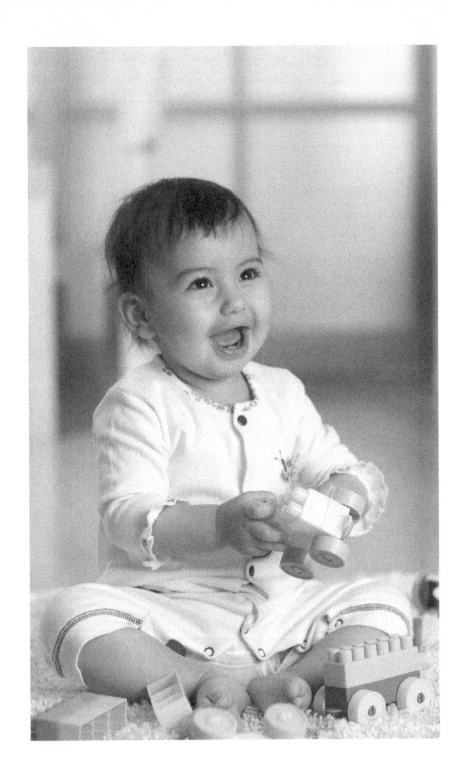

little annoying, but after a few goes you can just say, 'Okay, all done', and distract her with something else. What would you do without distractions!

At this age, she starts to be interested in pictures in a book for about a minute or so, but not the whole story. By 12 months, she can throw a toy.

You can see how fast she develops during this stage. You've come to understand how important you've been for her social, emotional and intellectual development. Through the first six months, you've lovingly fostered and nurtured her development by recognising and interpreting her non-verbal cues, facial expressions, her cries when she's upset and her emotions. Now she needs you to go with her to the next stage of her social, emotional and intellectual development, and that includes sharing your attention with the things she shows you she enjoys.

This is important because it helps her feel as if she's interesting and you're interested in her. Now she has the ability to spontaneously initiate little games, and invite you to join in with her. When you follow her lead, this builds her self-esteem and gives her the feeling that she can accomplish something. The game may be as simple as pat-a-cake or sharing a favourite toy.

Daily routine

Once again, your baby needs to have a predictable yet flexible routine that gives her a sense of security and certainty about her day. This will make her feel more relaxed during the day and help her to sleep better at night.

After 9 months, your baby's meals and bedtime routines will start to fit in more comfortably with the rest of the family. She may still wake early in the morning and she will need to go to bed early at night and have her daytime naps, but most of her sleep will be throughout the night-time hours and her meal schedule is simpler.

Sample routine for your 9- to 12-month-old baby

- Your baby may still wake at sunrise. Some babies still have an early morning milk feed, while others have discarded this feed (this is purely a personal choice). This is when she may start the day or return to sleep for a little while.
- Breakfast solids and a milk feed
- Playtime includes social time with you. She enjoys pulling toys with a string, dropping toys, poking things. She will babble to herself and shout to get your attention. She likes peek-a-boo and looking at books for about a minute.
- Going for a walk in the pram, visiting friends, baby playgroup
- Morning tea (perhaps fruit) and a drink of water
- Carefully watch your baby for when she gets drowsy and use your tired sign formula (see page 125). Remember, it's best to put her to bed when she's in a drowsy state.
- A nap of 1 to 2 hours
- Lunch solids and a milk feed
- Another playtime
- Carefully watch your baby for when she gets drowsy and use your tired sign formula (see page 125). Remember, it's best to put her to bed when she's in a drowsy state.
- A nap of 1 to 1½ hours
- Afternoon tea (perhaps fruit) and a drink of water
- Another playtime
- Dinner solids and a milk feed
- Quiet, wind-down cuddle time
- A bath and her bedtime routine and settle for the night
- She may still want one milk feed during the night.

Going to sleep between 6 and 12 months

Here you are in the second half of your baby's first year and maybe she still hasn't managed to either go to sleep on her own or go back to sleep when she wakes at night.

Or maybe your baby has reached 6 months and you thought she'd settled into a regular day–night sleep rhythm by now. She was mostly going to bed awake and able to soothe herself to sleep on most nights, and during awakenings was mostly able to self-settle. You were getting some sleep.

Then, she reached 6 months and something happened. Your baby suddenly started to wake frequently during the night again for no apparent reason. You don't know what's going on.

In Chapter 7, we looked at the two types of well-recognised sleep problems that occur over the first 12 months and can last into the toddler years:

1. Your baby has difficulties going to bed and falling asleep on her own.
2. Your baby can't return to sleep on her own after waking between sleep cycles.

It's believed there are the two possible reasons for why this happens:

1. Some babies' sleep development is more immature than other babies'. They need more help to fall asleep and also to go back to sleep when they wake between sleep cycles.
2. Other babies' sleep development may be maturing normally, but their parents might be so involved in putting their baby to sleep and are responding too quickly when their baby wakes during the night that their baby becomes reliant on this routine.

Now that your baby is 6 months and older, introduce soothing strategies that suit her developmental age. Tresillian uses a method called 'Responsive Settling'. (See Chapter 7 for information about Responsive Settling techniques for babies from birth to 6 months.)

Remember, Tresillian does not use controlled crying. Also, Tresillian follows Red Nose recommendations on safe sleeping for your baby to reduce the risk of Sudden Unexpected Deaths in Infancy (SUDI), including SIDS.

Responsive Settling: putting your baby to bed awake

To make sure you avoid resettling difficulties during the night, start the night by putting your baby to bed awake. This is a good time to begin with a simple, predictable bedtime routine.

Routine for putting your baby to bed awake

1. Begin with a cuddle and a soothing, calm bedtime routine.
2. Carefully watch your baby for when she gets drowsy and use your tired sign formula (see page 125). Remember, it's best to put her to bed when she's in a drowsy state.
3. Speak to her in a calm, soothing and low voice while you're getting her ready for bed and putting her into her bed. Sing her a lullaby if you enjoy singing.
4. Put her to sleep in the same familiar place as often as you can.
5. If it's daytime, you don't need to make the room totally dark – a little daylight is fine.
6. If it's night-time, ensure the light in the room isn't stimulating, such as light from the TV, computers, smartphones or tablets (see Chapter 1: How sleep works).
7. Give her a reassuring kiss or stroke her head and leave her to see if she can settle.

Responsive Settling: comfort settling technique

If your baby can't fall asleep on her own, use this technique to help her.

Comfort settling technique

1. Wrap your baby with her arms up on her chest so she can move them to her mouth if she needs to. Or use a sleeping bag with fitted armholes, and no hood (following Red Nose safe baby sleeping bag guidelines).
2. Talk quietly and cuddle your baby to help her to calm.
3. Put your baby on her back in her cot, awake and in a calm and drowsy state.
4. Comfort her with gentle 'shhh' sounds, rhythmic patting, rocking or stroking until she is calm or asleep.
5. As your baby calms or falls asleep, move away from her cot or leave the room.
6. If your baby starts to become distressed, return and comfort her using step 3 before moving away from her cot or leaving the room again.
7. You may have to repeat this several times before your baby is able to settle to sleep.
8. If your baby does not settle, pick her up and cuddle her until calm, then either:
   - re-attempt comfort settling
   - use the hands-on settling technique (see page 153)
   - get baby up and try again later.
9. As your baby learns to settle, it will take less time to calm.

Parental presence settling for babies over 6 months

You may prefer this option if your baby has never been separated from you at sleep time.

Parental presence settling technique

1. Talk quietly and cuddle your baby to help her to calm.
2. Put your baby on her back in her cot, awake and in a calm and drowsy state.
3. Comfort her with gentle 'shhh' sounds, rhythmic patting, rocking or stroking until she is calm or almost asleep.
4. Once your baby is calm, lie down or sit beside the cot within sight of her and pretend to be asleep.
5. If your baby remains awake, give a little cough or quietly say, 'Shhh, time to sleep', so she knows that you're still in the room.
6. If your baby becomes distressed, do the least amount to calm her. But you may need to do steps 1 to 3 again, then lie or sit beside her cot. You may have to repeat this several times before your baby is able to remain calm and become drowsy or fall asleep.
7. Stay in the room until your baby is asleep during the day and sleep in the same room with her during the night.
8. Continue this for at least one week or until she has three nights in a row of relatively uninterrupted sleep.
9. You can now begin to leave the room before your baby is asleep.

Unfortunately, on some days your baby will find it very difficult to settle. No matter what you try, it does not work. If you start to feel tired, frustrated, upset or anxious, it's likely that your baby will also remain upset and unsettled. If this happens, try to have some relaxation ideas up your sleeve, like slow and deep breathing or playing gentle music, to help you stay calm while settling your baby (see Chapter 3: The two sides of your sleep problems).

Sleep associations

If you are anxious that your baby is going to feel distressed, frightened or abandoned every time you put her to bed or when she wakes up between sleep cycles, this anxiety can become a difficulty for both of you and may cause sleep and settling problems.

Your baby can sense your anxiety, but she doesn't know what you're anxious about. All she senses from you is that something's wrong. Her instinct is to stay as close as she can to you, which can actually result in her being more difficult to settle to sleep. This can become a vicious cycle.

The thing is, if you're anxious that she might be distressed or frightened when she wakes between sleep cycles, you're going to go to her quickly to make sure she's okay. That's perfectly reasonable if she's really crying and calling for you, but sometimes she's not really crying and you still might go to check her.

A lot of the time she might just be making those normal little noises, such as a grunt, snort, sometimes a louder squeak or even a little call, and you may still interpret this as distress and go to see what's wrong. When you go to her too quickly, this doesn't give her a chance to have a good go at soothing herself to sleep.

As your baby grows older, she will be able to tolerate a small amount of frustration as she tries to soothe herself to sleep, but not too much.

She will let you know when it's getting too hard for her. Remember that the attempt to self-settle is important for her development.

The difficulty of thinking your baby is distressed when she's actually making small noises in between a sleep cycle is that you might pick her up, feed her or rock her, when really she just needs to be left to see if she will resettle herself. These noises are not a sign that she's distressed: she's not actually crying or fussing.

When she becomes used to you being so actively involved in putting her to sleep, she begins to rely on you to go to sleep. She associates you and your method of putting her to sleep with going to sleep.

As we looked at briefly in the previous chapter, these are called 'sleep associations', which means that whatever you do to put your baby to sleep, such as feed her or hold her until she's asleep, becomes a pattern she will expect each time she wakes up, even throughout the night, to help her go back to sleep.

These constant interruptions throughout the night not only affect your sleep, but they affect hers as well. If you feel grumpy and tired, she will too. She's not much different from you really. Broken sleep affects you both in the same way.

It's quite possible that you know all this, but you still find it really hard to stop feeding your baby to sleep, holding her in your arms to put her to sleep, putting her in your bed, rocking her, driving around the block and all the other weird and wonderful things parents do to try to get their baby to sleep.

The trouble is, you will both develop a habit and, like any habit, it can be difficult to break. It's hard enough to break your own habit, but you will also be trying to break your sweet little baby's habit, and she has no desire to stop feeding, rocking, sleeping in your arms or any other comfy stuff you've been doing. Originally, these may have been positive sleep associations when your baby was very young, but now they may no longer be helpful for either of you.

Changing unhelpful sleep associations

If you think that some of this applies to you, here are some ideas you can try:

- Recognise the sleep associations you're using when you put your baby to bed at night and back to sleep during the night.
- When trying to change any sleep associations that have become unhelpful, you might find using Tresillian's Responsive Settling techniques for babies over 6 months helpful (see pages 170–2).
- Listen to the sounds your baby is making and try to interpret when she's genuinely distressed and you need to respond to her fussing or crying (see Chapter 5: Why your baby cries).
- Remind yourself that when your baby wakes between sleep cycles and makes normal little noises that mean she's trying to self-soothe, you need to wait and listen to see if she can go back to sleep on her own. This means holding off going to her for a few moments.
- Recognise your own distress when she wakes and is trying to self-soothe. You may be going to her too quickly because you're worried. You need to self-soothe as well! Reassure yourself, take a deep breath and hold yourself back until you're certain she needs your help.

Crawling

What an achievement! Your baby is finally able to move on her own!

Crawling is one of the most momentous milestones your baby can reach, and it usually begins sometime between 5 to 10 months. Imagine, you have never been able to move around without help and suddenly you can get somewhere on your own! The world is your oyster.

But for some babies, the achievement of crawling brings drawbacks when it comes to sleep. Here's what can happen:

- When your baby wakes at night, instead of soothing herself she may wake more fully and sit up or crawl around her cot. This could make her confused and anxious, especially in the dark.
- When she's more alert and awake, she's less able to soothe herself back to sleep. This means she's more likely to call out or even cry for your help to get back to sleep.

Why would this happen? It's thought that with the achievement of major developmental and intellectual milestones, your baby has a short period of unpredictability while she gets used to the big changes her body and brain are going through. So when she has a major growth spurt in one area, another area of her development that was perfectly fine may be affected. This can be confusing for both of you.

You are so proud of your baby because she is starting to crawl. You take photos and share the news, but suddenly she starts to wake every 2 hours at night again! What happened there? It's just another part of your baby's normal development; a step forward with a big achievement and a little step back with a sleep disruption as she gets used to her new body and her new way of thinking about her world.

As with any sleep disruption, it's time to use some gentle and reassuring settling strategies to help her over this developmental hump.

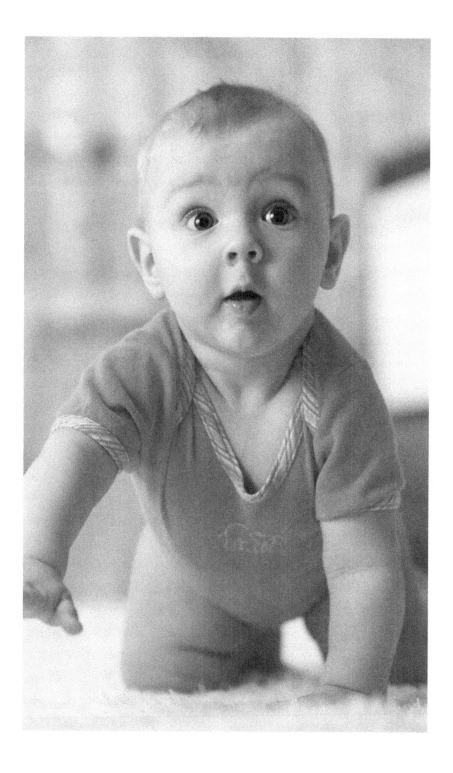

Separation anxiety

When she's 6 to 8 months of age, your baby will totally fall in love with you. Prior to this, even though she preferred you to anyone she would probably have been happy to talk to most people, but now you're her favourite person in the whole world. When she separates from you or you're out of her sight, she becomes anxious. She may cry and fret for you. Before she was 6 months old she really didn't know if you still existed when you left her, now she knows that when you leave the room you are somewhere else. So, she will definitely protest if you try to leave her.

Some babies have greater separation anxiety than others and that's thought to be due to a combination of things, such as their personality, temperament, relationships and what's going on in their households.

Your baby may have been able to self-settle to sleep quite well prior to the development of separation anxiety, but it does have the potential to affect her sleep because sleep involves a separation from you. She has to go to bed and separate from her treasured parent, special toys and exciting household goings-on. When she wakes from her sleep, it's dark and she's alone. Instead of soothing herself back to sleep, she remembers you're somewhere in the house.

For her, this is the time to see you again. It doesn't matter if it's not morning yet – from her standpoint she wants to be together with you again. This is when your baby will call out to you or, if she's been awake for a while, she may start to cry.

If your baby suddenly experiences a period of separation anxiety where she cries and calls for you at night and is unable to self-settle, then in this case, she does need you to respond to her promptly. When she's crying, go to her and reassure, calm and soothe her. Once you've done that, you can try to resettle her back to sleep. You can use the Tresillian Responsive Settling techniques to help you resettle her. You may have to keep using the settling techniques until this developmental phase passes.

Separation anxiety doesn't just belong to your baby. You can feel a certain amount of it as well. You have a natural response to your baby calling out and crying, especially at night-time, when it's dark. You want to go to her and protect her – it's natural. Human beings don't like darkness and being alone because our primitive instincts tell us it's dangerous. A small amount of separation anxiety is totally natural, but if you experience a great deal of separation anxiety when your baby wakes at night and can't soothe herself back to sleep, you could go back to Chapter 3: The two sides of your sleep problems, and read about anxiety and some strategies to help you to calm down before you go to help her.

During the second half of her first year, your baby is rapidly changing as she becomes more mobile and her relationship with you deepens and grows. These changes affect many aspects of her development, including her sleep. The physical, social and emotional changes are both wonderful and exciting, but they can also be a bit confusing.

As difficult, tiring and disappointing as some of these setbacks are, you now know there are reasons why her sleep gets disrupted. There's usually nothing wrong with your baby, she's probably just going through her normal developmental changes.

Theresa's story (mother of Madeleine, 22 months)

Madeleine was always one of those babies who couldn't settle on her own. From the very beginning, she didn't like to be put down and always wanted to be held and rocked to sleep. We knew this was normal in the first few months, so we spent a lot of time holding her and cuddling her. Every nap I would rock or feed her to sleep and initially I was okay with that. She was happy and thriving, and that was all that mattered.

However, the months went on and I still couldn't get her to sleep without rocking her. Every time I would put her in her cot when she was awake, she would scream until I picked her up. She couldn't even be drowsy; she had to be absolutely fast asleep for me to put her down.

There was a period when she was waking up after 30 minutes during the day and sometimes every 40 minutes at night. It was just ridiculous – I was getting absolutely no rest and was a complete mess.

I went to Tresillian Day Services when she was about 9 months old. The nurses gave me some other techniques to try and settle her. They advised the parental presence technique, where I put her down in the cot, then lay on the floor and pretended to sleep so she felt reassured enough to go to sleep. I have to say, it certainly didn't happen overnight. It took a month or two of persisting and we often had to pick her up and cuddle her before putting her down and starting again. But gradually she got used to the new routine and started to go to sleep pretty quickly.

At night, she was still waking frequently but then all of a sudden, she slept through. Then the next night she did it again and the night after that. She was about 10 months old at the time and she now sleeps through every night except when she's sick. It's just amazing! She still likes me to be there when she falls asleep, but I don't mind giving her that reassurance when I know I'm going to get a full night's sleep.

It was a really tough road but, in hindsight, I wish I hadn't worried as much about having a child who didn't sleep through the night. I believe that Madeleine just wanted to be near me and wasn't ready yet to spend all night without me. When she was developmentally ready, she slept. For us, it was as simple as that.

Key message

- During this second six months, your baby's sleep patterns usually change very little. She will continue to sleep continuously for stretches of about 5 to 6 hours a night on most nights and wake two to three times.
- It's thought that with the achievement of major developmental and intellectual milestones, such as crawling, your baby has a short period of unpredictability while she gets used to the big changes her body and brain are going through.
- Remind yourself that when your baby wakes between sleep cycles and makes normal little noises that mean she's trying to self-soothe, you need to give her the chance to self-settle. Rather than going to her too quickly, wait and listen to see if she can go back to sleep on her own.

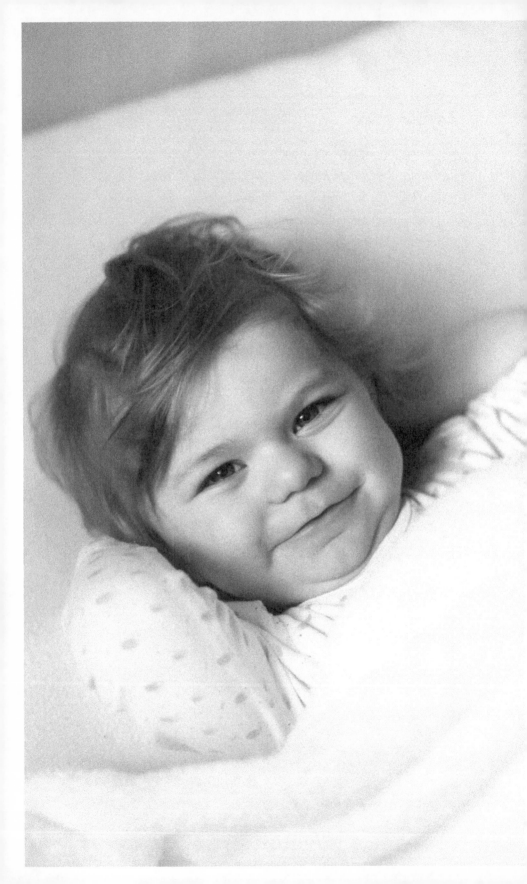

CHAPTER 9

Your toddler and sleep: 12 to 36 months

Well, you're there! Your baby has reached 12 months and she's pretty much a toddler. Unfortunately, toddlers get a lot of bad media coverage – they have been described as 'terrible' for so long now that people believe it to be true.

Words are powerful, and when people call someone 'terrible', they are apt to believe it and treat them that way. It's important to reflect on the way you think and talk about your toddler. If you unconsciously expect your toddler to be terrible, how will you treat her? And how does the way you think about her affect your approach to these important years of her life?

Understanding your toddler's behaviour

Your toddler lives in the moment. There is no 'just wait a minute' for her. Every single little thing is fascinating right now. This makes your toddler very interesting and a real joy to be with when she's exploring and sharing all her discoveries with you.

She has such enormous fun with simple activities like splashing in water, swishing her hand in dirt and poking her fingers into whatever she can find, no matter how dangerous it is. A single leaf is fascinating and probably needs to be tasted as well as handled, smelled and looked at.

Discovery and delight in the world are her business. If you join in with her, you can also rediscover splashing water, the beauty of leaves and watching ants march along the path.

There is no 'just wait a minute'
for your toddler. Every single little
thing is fascinating right now.

Your toddler is so intent on single-minded discovery that she can't wait when you want to dress her. You're interrupting her. She doesn't understand about waiting because she lives for now.

So, what happens when you interrupt her to get dressed, eat her lunch or get in the car? Sadly, this is when you see the side of your toddler that everyone focuses on – her frustration and annoyance. She can't tell you in words that she hasn't finished exploring and investigating, so she'll tell you with emotions and non-verbal cues.

First, she'll give you small signals, such as ignore you, look away from you, shake her head or look down and keep playing. When you insist and go to pick her up, you'll get the emotional eruption of pulling away, crying, kicking, back arching – the dreaded tantrum. You will always get small signals prior to a major tantrum.

However, put yourself in her place and imagine if you only lived in the moment. Even if the interruption to what you're doing takes just 5 minutes of your time, this doesn't mean a thing to you. What does matter is that all the fun has disappeared from this moment. Getting dressed or eating lunch would seem like forever, so you would probably get upset and angry. You would probably need someone to help you sort out your feelings and calm down.

Your toddler needs this as well, and the small signals are your warning signs. She needs some extra help with getting ready for changes when she's involved in voyages of discovery. Your toddler has to manage mundane, everyday activities, so you have to calculate that into your flexible daily routine.

There's no doubt that your toddler is absolutely delightful one minute and will drive you crazy the next. She can be unpredictable, disruptive and seem to repeat the same behaviour over and over again.

There was a meme travelling social media that described most toddlers beautifully: 'Hell hath no fury like a toddler whose sandwich has been cut into squares when she wanted triangles.'

The reality of that problem is that you can't do anything about it. Your toddler doesn't have the ability to tell you that today is triangle day. Apart from not knowing what a triangle is, how could she? She doesn't have the words. She may not have known that she wanted triangles until you gave her squares. That's because she lives in the moment. It can be a confusing time for you both.

It's tempting in this situation to argue with her, but don't bother arguing with your toddler over things you can't possibly win. It's exhausting and frustrating, and you just won't enjoy your relationship with each other. She may also have lots more tantrums because she will be frustrated as well.

What you can do

Leave her with her sandwich squares and if she has a tantrum, help her through her toddler dilemma by understanding her disappointment. Stay with her until she comes to terms with squares.

Or simply make another sandwich and cut it into triangles.

The main point about this dilemma is that the battle of wills over eating the sandwich, or any other food you have lovingly made, isn't worth fighting about. What your toddler puts in her mouth and swallows and eliminates out of her body is completely under her control. You will never win that battle. In fact, it can become a power game that you can't win, so don't even try.

Use your limit-setting for important things like ensuring she's safe, such as making sure she doesn't touch power points or run away from you – that sort of thing.

When your toddler displays the same behaviour over and over again, it can be so annoying and infuriating. You seem to be saying 'No!' a hundred times a day. She's not really being naughty, you know. She just forgets what she can't do. There are a lot of rules to learn and her brain isn't quite able to remember them all yet. And besides, everything is so interesting.

When she goes to touch a power point or play with the dirt in a pot plant or open the kitchen cupboard and turns to look at you, sometimes smiling before she touches it, she's checking with you. She's asking, 'Remind me, did you tell me I'm not supposed to touch this or do that?'

She's not being naughty or defiant. With your constant help, she is learning how to control her impulse to touch what you don't want her to touch. The way you do this is to gently and firmly say 'no' and then pick her up, turn her around and give her something else to do. You might have to do that a hundred times. At this age, you have to distract her while you teach her to follow your instructions to not touch dangerous things.

Yes, this is irritating. But eventually, her memory of your calm and helpful instructions will start to have an impact. She'll understand she can't touch certain things, recognise that you mean 'no' and learn to control her impulses. And that will help her at day care, preschool and school. She'll have a better learning experience when she can control her impulses and understand there are certain things that she can't do when she's told 'no'.

With this type of gentle, consistent help from you, by 3 years of age she may be able to control her impulses for a minute, take a turn and share toy and, best of all, will sometimes cooperate with you and her friends.

As for her tantrums, your toddler won't learn how to manage her big out-of-control feelings by being put into time out. She needs your help to calm down, the same as she did when she was a young baby (see Chapter 5: Why your baby cries).

Imagine what it's like when you're extremely upset and need comforting. You usually like someone to comfort you or at least acknowledge you're upset. But if everyone around you totally ignores your distress and need for help, that feels awful.

Your toddler is exactly the same, except it's even worse for her. She needs lots of help to manage her out-of-control feelings of anger, frustration and disappointment. She doesn't even understand yet that these are the emotions she's feeling.

If you would like to know more about managing tantrums and why time out isn't a useful method for toddlers and young children, visit the website of the Australian Association for Infant Mental Health Inc (aaimhi.org) and read their position paper on time out.

During her second year, your toddler is rapidly developing physically, intellectually, emotionally and socially. She loves to explore and this means moving away from you more and more. But she has a dilemma because she needs to stay close to you as well, and that creates some tension because she wants to be a little independent now. This can get a bit complicated for her, because at about 18 months she may have another episode of separation anxiety. She wants to stay close to you, but she desperately wants to use her new skills of crawling and walking to get away from you and explore.

You just have to gently balance her two opposing needs: to stay close to you and have cuddles, while also gaining a little independence to explore. Once again, this can be confusing for her. She wants to get up on your lap and then pushes you away and struggles to get down; then, she may go through the whole performance again. She's also resentful of other children and sometimes very demanding of your attention!

187

This is normal toddler development that's not well understood, and it's confusing for both of you. Your toddler isn't being difficult, naughty or terrible – she's just a bit hard to work out sometimes. Throughout these 12 to 36 months, your toddler is still socially and emotionally dependent on you and needs plenty of reassurance as she learns to manage a complicated social world.

Your toddler's emotional and intellectual world

Your toddler is a very emotional person, and, at times, she's unable to manage or control her emotions. She relies on your help.

Her emotions drive her behaviour. Your toddler has a tantrum because she's upset, angry or frustrated. Something happened to bring her to that emotional state, so it makes sense to figure out what happened prior to the tantrum to cause the emotion, and try to prevent it from happening again, if you can.

A good example is biting or hitting. Your toddler doesn't just bite or hit for any reason, there are always two (or more) people involved in interactions.

She may bite or hit because she's angry, so you need to find out what happened that made her angry. A situation occurs, usually with a playmate, that causes an emotion, such as frustration or anger, and then the behaviour happens. It helps to understand if you can find out what happened between the toddlers that led to the situation that caused the bite or hit to occur. There's always an emotion that drives your toddler's behaviour.

Emotions drive your behaviour as well, it's just that you know what feelings you're having and you can usually do something about them. Your toddler can't understand or put a name to her feelings yet, so she needs your help to figure out her feelings and for you to name them for her. She also needs you to help her control her impulses because she can't do that either.

When you're really unable to help her, it's time for you to sit down, count to three and use some deep breathing exercises (see page 55). This will help you calm down before you begin to try to figure out what your toddler is up to now.

Sometimes when you're really tired, it's almost impossible to manage your feelings, let alone your toddler's, and you might even wonder why on earth you thought being a parent was a good idea! Don't worry, all parents feel like that from time to time.

As Charles Dickens wrote a long time ago, 'It was the best of times, it was the worst of times'. He was writing about the French Revolution, but his words could just as easily be applied to parenting a toddler.

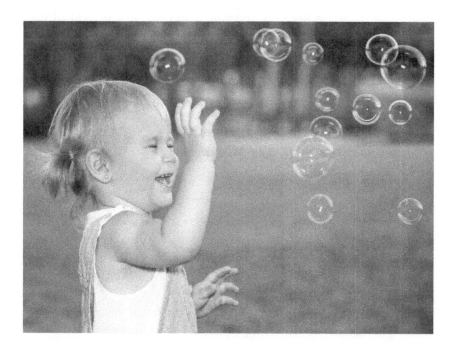

Toddler routines

During her second year, your toddler's meals and bedtime routines fit more comfortably into the rest of the family's. From 12 to 18 months she may still wake early in the morning, but as she gets closer to 2 years she may sleep later in the morning. At 2½ to 3 years old, she will more closely sync with your family routines. She will begin to imitate you, say some words and use a spoon to feed herself. She will still need to go to bed fairly early at night and most of her sleep will be throughout the night-time hours.

Her daytime naps will get shorter. She may still have two naps a day by the time she reaches 18 months old, one longer one and a short catnap. Between 18 months and 3 years, naps reduce to about 1 to 2 hours. But remember, your toddler is an individual and her own individual sleep rhythms determine her sleep requirements.

Sample routine for your toddler

- Your toddler usually wakes at sunrise.
- At 12 to 14 months, your toddler still has an early morning milk feed, but as she gets older she may discard it. This is purely a personal choice. Once again, this is when she may start the day or may return to sleep for a little while.
- From 18 months, your toddler may still want a milk feed from the breast, bottle or cup, or simply be ready for breakfast as soon as she gets up. This will also depend on you and when you want to wean your toddler from the breast or bottle.
- By 3 years old, most toddlers will be fitting in with the family meal times.
- Breakfast

- Playtime includes social time with you, toys and games
- Going for a walk, visiting friends, playgroup
- Morning tea (possibly fruit) and a drink of water
- She may have a morning nap of 1 to 2 hours.
- Carefully watch your toddler for when she gets drowsy and use your tired sign formula (see page 125). Remember, it's best to put her to bed when she's in a drowsy state.
- Lunch solids and a milk feed
- Another playtime
- She may have an afternoon nap of 1 to 2 hours. Her naps may start to change from 18 months and she may only have one nap of 2 hours each day. She may nap during the day until she is about 3 years old.
- Carefully watch your toddler for when she gets drowsy and use your tired sign formula (see page 125). Remember, it's best to put her to bed when she's in a drowsy state.
- Afternoon tea (possibly fruit) and a drink of water
- Another playtime
- Dinner solids and a milk feed from the breast or bottle, depending on her age
- Quiet, wind-down cuddle time
- A bath and her soothing bedtime routine
- Your toddler is ready for books with pictures. She'll enjoy turning the pages and listening to you make animal noises. At 2½ years, her attention span is longer and she can focus more on her books and point to small, interesting details.
- Once her bedtime routine is over, settle her for the night.
- At 12 to 14 months, she may still want one milk feed overnight. After this age, she doesn't need to feed at night.

Respond to her tired signs by
reducing stimulation and adopting
a calm and soothing presence.

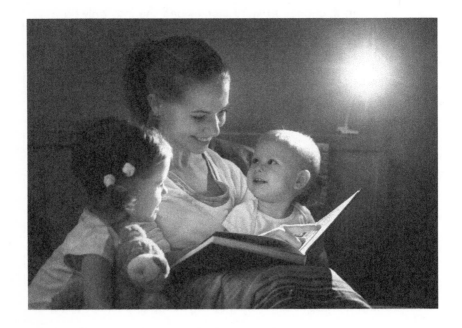

The tired signs for a toddler

When your toddler becomes tired or overtired, the most important sign to look for is drowsiness plus one or more of the following non-verbal cues.

Toddler tired signs

- drowsiness
- heavy eyelids and glazed, dull eyes
- yawning
- still, quiet, not very alert
- irritable, restless
- clumsiness
- grizzling, fussy
- sucking her thumb or a dummy, if she uses one
- searching for her special blanket, toy or comforter.

Respond to her tired signs by reducing stimulation and adopting a calm and soothing presence. She needs you to tell her she's tired so that she can begin to understand what it feels like to be tired, and that this feeling means she needs to go to bed and have a sleep.

Once you have noticed she's tired and ready for a sleep, prepare your toddler for going to bed. The bedtime routine you use will depend on the time of day and her age. For example, if it's a daytime nap you might simply put the toys away, talk to her quietly, pick her up and give her a cuddle, then move on to a short, quiet, calming and predictable bedtime routine to help her wind down and get ready to lie down in her cot or bed, depending on her age. If it's night time, close the curtains in her room and turn off the lights (see Chapter 1: How sleep works).

For her first 12 months, you may have had a familiar, predictable bedtime routine for your baby. Now that your toddler's day fits more closely to the family's routines, she will definitely need a comforting routine each evening that signals that it's the end of the day and time for her long night-time sleep. This will give her time to wind down, relax with you and get ready for bed and sleep. The same, familiar, calming bedtime routine will usually result in her falling asleep more quickly and may also reduce any anxiety or disruptive behaviours at this time.

Night-time routines usually include a bath. Even though baths are fun, they are always warm and relaxing; you know yourself how a bath feels. Routines include a nappy change, teeth cleaning, cuddles and a quiet story together, and tucking in or placing her in a sleeping bag, depending on her age. Some parents and toddlers have a favourite quiet song they like to sing at bedtime.

These quiet wind-down routines are always followed by moving your toddler into her cot or bed and an affectionate kiss goodnight. Your toddler thrives on your affection. Her brain grows stronger and healthy neural connections are made every time you touch her, gently kiss her and tell her you love her.

If your toddler has chosen a special blanket, toy or comforter, she will need this as part of her bedtime routine. At around or after the stage when your baby experiences separation anxiety, she will choose the blanket or toy that will become her special comforter. It's thought that the special object your baby chooses provides her with comfort and security in your absence. That's why this object is so important to her when she separates from you to go to bed and to help her calm down when she gets upset. No one can choose this object for her, this is something she has to choose for herself.

Once you have finished your routine and your toddler is drowsy and ready for sleep, put her into her cot or bed awake, kiss her goodnight and leave her to fall asleep.

Always ensure that the cot sides are up and securely in place.

When your toddler won't settle

Here are some Tresillian settling strategies to try if your toddler still has difficulties going to sleep on her own and wakes through the night.

Toddler settling strategies

- If you have tried putting your toddler to bed and she continues to be distressed or she's crying, pick her up and cuddle her until she's calm. And check her nappy. You can then attempt to resettle her.
- Speak gently and quietly to reassure her, such as telling her, 'It's time for sleep'. You want to encourage a state of calm. Once she's calm again, position her comfortably on her back in her cot or bed while she's still awake.
- If she still doesn't respond and she cries, pick her up again and cuddle her until she's calm.
- You could try giving her a drink of water but nothing else.
- If she's very upset, then try staying in the room until she falls asleep. You could sit on a chair quietly. The length of time it takes to calm your toddler will decrease as she begins to calm herself and self-settles to sleep.
- If you find your toddler needs you to stay in the room while she falls asleep, try sitting on a chair beside her cot or her bed, and then, over time, gradually move your chair a little further away as she gains more confidence in her ability to fall asleep without you being quite so close. Eventually, move your chair until you are sitting near or just outside the door, responding to her with your gentle voice if she checks that you're still there. You might like to try the parental presence settling technique in Chapter 8 (see page 172) if your toddler is anxious about separating from you at sleep time.

Transitioning from cot to regular bed

If your toddler is starting to climb out of her cot or onto the cot sides, it's time to transition from a cot to a regular bed. Moving into a bed is an exciting step in your child's life and some of these points may help to smooth out any problems the move may make.

Transitioning to a regular bed

1. Start by encouraging her to climb into her bed unaided.

2. Give your toddler verbal reassurances and tell her what's going to happen next, such as 'It's bedtime now'. In a calm, firm voice give positive instructions like, 'It's time to go to sleep', to discourage her from climbing out of bed.

3. In the early days, keep a familiar blanket or toy your toddler chooses from her cot to help make her feel more secure in her new bed. If she has a special blanket or toy, she'll take that with her. Remember to check that any comfort object she takes to bed with her is safe, with nothing that she could swallow or choke on.

4. Praise your toddler if she manages to stay in her 'big bed'!

5. If she does get out of bed, gently and firmly walk her back to bed, tuck her in again and say goodnight. Sometimes you have to do that a few times and, as annoying as it is, it's best to stay as calm as possible until she gets the idea.

6. If need be, use the settling techniques we have looked at, such as sitting beside the bed and over time moving your chair gradually further away, until your toddler gets used to going to sleep in her new bed.

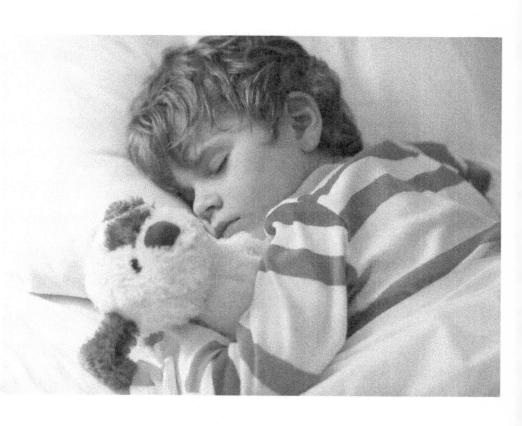

Your toddler is a delightful little person most of the time. The more you watch her, figure out her non-verbal cues and understand that she lives in the moment, the more her behaviour will make sense to you.

When you're stuck trying to figure out what your toddler is doing, put yourself in her place and ask, 'What would that be like for me?'

Imagine having:

- a very limited alibility to speak or understand your language
- no experience of crawling or walking
- just the beginnings of the ability to manage or even know what emotions you're feeling
- strong emotions that are so out of control they scare you
- no sense of time
- difficulty in understanding that other people have needs or feelings different to yours
- the urge to explore and discover everything but someone always seems to stop you
- very little control over anything in your world
- so much excitement you want to share with your favourite people right this minute – everything else can wait.

Your toddler must have a strange, wonderful but, very often, frustrating life. From your point of view, she is light and dark! One moment she's a total delight and then exhausting and frustrating the next. But she's never terrible. That's just bad media coverage that toddlers have been getting for too long.

Your toddler will need a lot of help in managing her world. When you figure out what's bothering her and help her sort it out, your life becomes much more peaceful – well, most of the time.

Mia's story (mother of William, 2½ years, and Anna, 3 months)

William was 14 months old when we went to Tresillian Residential. At the time, he was still waking at least three or four times a night. I was really struggling to break some of his habits, like still having night-time bottles.

There were a few reasons why it had become so bad. He was still sleeping in our room at that stage because we had the only air-conditioning unit in the house. When we tried to put him in his own room, he had a habit of getting hysterical and vomiting. As he was over 12 months, he had become so much more aware and dependent on us being there. Some of the habits he'd formed were really hard to break.

At Tresillian, we learned how to reset the rules. First of all, we found out that he needed to eat more food during the day in order to sustain him overnight. We were giving him meals but the portions were probably too small and we hadn't been giving him snacks, so we started to increase all the sizes and add more variety.

Next, we had to teach him that being in a cot in his own room was okay. My husband and I had really different ideas of how to settle him, so it was really helpful being given consistent support from the nurses on the best way to do it. When William woke, the nurses would sit with us as we listened to his cries. If he vomited, we would go in and change him, then calm him down before putting him back in his cot. We would shush him a bit, then leave the room. We kept doing that, leaving the room to give him an opportunity to build confidence in settling himself, and returning to comfort him, until, eventually, he went to sleep.

After that first night, we saw an 80 per cent improvement and, by the end of the week, he was sleeping through the night. It was just incredible! I'm so thankful for the nurses and I'm really proud of William for breaking the cycle.

It's more than a year later now, and he's still sleeping through the night almost every night. I've recently had a new baby and I'm determined not to repeat any of those mistakes with this one. I've already been putting her down awake, but calm, to help her learn to self-settle and so far it's working well.

The main thing I've learned is that it's okay for them to grizzle a little for the greater outcome of getting them to self-settle. I just wish I'd received some help earlier. I think anyone who is struggling should just go and get help rather than trying to do it themselves.

Key message

- Your toddler has to manage mundane, everyday activities, so you have to calculate that into your flexible daily routine. Use your limit-setting for important things like ensuring she's safe, such as making sure she doesn't touch power points or run away from you.
- During her second and third years, your toddler's meals and bedtime routines fit more comfortably into the rest of the family's.
- Once your toddler starts to climb out of her cot, it's time for her to transition to a 'big bed'. This is an exciting experience for her, but it may take time and encouragement to keep her in her new big bed at night. This means you'll need to remain calm and reassuring as well as use settling techniques to help her settle to sleep.

CHAPTER 10

Your preschooler and sleep: 3 to 5 years

At 3 years old, your toddler has grown into a preschooler. From 3 to 5 years, she will spend about half her day asleep, most of it at night if she doesn't have daytime naps. If she does have daytime naps, she will still have the same amount of sleep per day, but she'll probably go to bed later in the evening. During these years, the average amount of sleep she will need each day is about 10 to 12 hours.

Your preschooler's sleep can be affected by various things, including many of the issues we looked at in the previous chapters. Additionally, she is venturing into the world and socialising more with her peers and other adults. Although this can be fun and exciting, she has a lot to cope with socially and emotionally and this can also impact on her sleep. It's important to understand your preschooler's development when you think about reasons for why she might be having sleeping difficulties.

Who your preschooler is

During these preschool years, she continues to develop physically, mentally, socially and emotionally. Note that her social and emotional development is most important in preparation for her formal school years.

Research has shown that your child's ability to do well at school, enjoy satisfying friendships and have good relationships with her teachers depends more on her ability to manage her emotions than her ability to write her name and know her numbers prior to starting kindergarten.

By socialising more with her peers and new adults, your preschooler will have a lot to cope with socially and emotionally.

'Why is this?' you might ask. 'Doesn't everyone say it's really important to teach my child to read and count to be ready for school?'

Well, the answer is 'no'. Your preschooler can go to school unable to write her name or count and yet still catch up if she can sit quietly and focus on the task at hand. However, if your child can't sit still and focus on the task the teacher gives her, if she cries or gets angry because the teacher makes her sit still, then she isn't going to be happy or in an emotional state to be able to focus and learn.

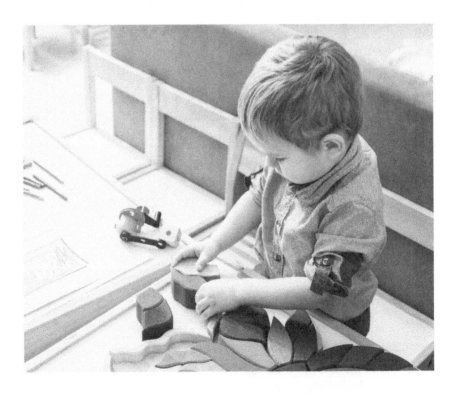

If she hasn't learned to wait her turn in a game or share toys with other children, becomes angry or frustrated and can't manage her anger with the other children, she may have difficulties with her friends at preschool, and later at school. And this might make her sad.

If she's unable to socialise well or manage to control her emotions, it doesn't matter if she can write her name or count. In such an unhappy and difficult environment, she may begin to feel bad about herself, her learning may suffer and so may her behaviour.

During these early years, her social and emotional development is crucial. You may not have realised it, but right from birth you've been helping her manage her emotions and preparing her for school. These are some of the ways you have helped her cope with her emotions so she could begin to gain some control over them. You:

- carried and calmed her as a baby during the peak stage of crying and at other times she cried
- played games with her, smiled, touched her and showed her lots of affection
- had a calm, soothing routine for when she was upset, from babyhood through toddlerhood
- helped her manage the big emotions that she couldn't handle herself throughout babyhood and toddlerhood
- used sleep and settling strategies that helped her self-soothe
- recognised her non-verbal cues and responded when she needed a break or needed to play
- had a relaxed, flexible and predictable daily routine
- had a calm and soothing bedtime routine
- helped your baby and toddler to focus and enjoy stories or games for short periods of time by following her lead.

Your preschooler's social-emotional world

Let's look at what sort of emotional development is happening through the preschool years and how can you continue to help her manage her emotions.

During these preschool years, she continues to develop her ability to focus on activities for longer periods of time. To be able to focus she has to resist her impulse to get distracted by other interesting activities. This is quite difficult for her and she may sometimes need your help.

She is also learning to solve problems with your help and guidance, as well as stopping herself from doing something you tell her not to do. This is learning self-control, which is very important for transitioning to school.

When she was a toddler, you might have started naming her feelings when she was upset. If you did that, she will now start to use words to name and describe her feelings. When she recognises her own feelings, she's more likely to empathise with other people. This is a wonderful quality to have and will help her at school and throughout life.

Once she's able to name her
emotions and start to manage
them, she'll begin to recognise the
same emotions in other people.

Once she's able to name her emotions and start to manage them, she'll begin to recognise the same emotions in other people. If you have helped her manage the big emotions of toddlerhood, she'll start to manage her negative feelings, such as her anger and frustration. She will be able to tell you with her own words how angry, sad or happy she is.

She'll still need your help sometimes with anger or over-excitement. When she does need your help, you can revert back to the ways you assisted her when she was a toddler. Remember, it's hard to be grown up all the time, especially when she's tired or sick.

What you can do

If you are not seeing some of these developmental changes in your preschooler, here are some suggestions on ways to help her get on track with her social and emotional development.

Helping your preschooler manage her emotions

- If you haven't already, begin naming her feelings and describing what she's feeling. Help and support her to calm down when she's angry, frustrated, scared, overexcited or disruptive. Sometimes, she may be disruptive because she's angry or frustrated and she just doesn't know what she's feeling. That's why she needs you to remain calm and support her to calm down. This may be hard at first and it may take a little time to get back on track.

- If you are already noticing and naming her emotions, continue to do so. You can also name your own feelings, but be careful not to give her too much detail about why you're feeling angry or sad. At this age, she's unable to understand adult problems and you could make her anxious.

- If she has tantrums and you use time out as a method, this may not be working for her. If she is alone during the time out, no one is with her to help and support her to calm down. She may not understand what she is feeling or why she has been separated from you when she's upset.

This method of time out may not help her when she goes to school, as she won't know how to calm down on her own or be able to use her words to explain her feelings. She may have to leave the classroom to calm down if she's disruptive.

If you would like to know more about managing tantrums and concerns about the use of time out for young children, visit the website of the Australian Association for Infant Mental Health Inc (aaimhi.org).

Trying to reason with your preschooler when she's angry, frustrated and upset is pointless. Trying to reason with adults when they're upset usually doesn't work either, so it definitely won't work with your preschooler. Chances are you may feel quite upset, too.

At this age, your child is developing her capacity to think and problem-solve. So, once you've both calmed down, sit together and think about what happened that caused her to get angry. This is an opportunity to talk about how your preschooler can manage the same difficult situation next time, such as a toy set not working properly, or her baby brother wrecking a game. Continuing to do this through her preschool years will get her ready to cope with difficult social and emotional situations later at school.

- If you haven't already established calm, predictable, yet flexible daily and bedtime routines, now is the time to start. Your preschooler will enjoy knowing what to expect during the day and as bedtime approaches (see sample routines on pages 209–10).
- Play with your preschooler. Ask her what she enjoys doing, encourage her to choose the game and then let her be in charge of it. Get down on the floor with her and follow her lead. Watch her carefully and, if you think she needs your help, ask her before stepping in and taking over.

If she does accept your help, work with her and make suggestions, rather than doing it for her. Help her problem-solve by saying things like, 'Do you think it could go another way?' or 'What about that piece?', rather than saying, 'Put it there' or 'Do it like this'. Tell her how well she's doing. Encouraging her and making suggestions helps her to feel she's done something successfully on her own. That's a nice feeling.

She loves to be praised. The best type of praise to give her is to tell her the behaviour that pleases you, right at the moment she does it. That way she knows exactly what to do. Give her gentle praise each time she:

- uses her words when she's angry
- waits her turn in a game with you or her friends
- shares her toys
- listens and follows your directions.

> The best type of praise to give her is to tell her the behaviour that pleases you, right at the moment she does it.

You don't have to get out the confetti cannon every time you praise her, though. It's not like she's displaying some sort of superhero power – you're just helping her to develop and manage her social and emotional skills. Simple, positive feedback, such as 'Good listening' or 'Good sharing', is all she needs to help her understand she's doing well developing her social and emotional skills.

If she's having difficulties with controlling her impulses, try playing games like:

- stop dancing when the music stops
- Simon Says
- Red Light – Green Light.

Work on her not interrupting you. For example, ask her to wait until you finish talking to someone – just for a brief moment. You can also practice waiting together. This can be for anything, like baking a cake or waiting in a queue.

- If she has trouble with taking turns, play turn-taking games that she can practice with you. Help her learn to manage her frustration while she waits.

Preschooler routines and sleep needs

For the most part, your preschooler will fit in with the family's routines. She's able to eat meals with the rest of the family and enjoy the same food. She will still need to go to bed fairly early at night and most of her sleep will be throughout the night-time hours. She will need about 10 to 12 hours of sleep a day, and this includes both her day and night sleep.

Your preschooler may not have a daytime nap every day, although if she goes to long day-care, she will probably be encouraged to have a rest or sleep once a day. Having a day sleep can sometimes push her bedtime back till later because she still only needs the same number of hours of sleep every 24 hours. So, be prepared for a later bedtime if you like your child to take naps or if she needs them.

If she does have a nap, it will probably be anywhere from 50 minutes to 1½ hours, depending on how tired she is. Once again, your child is an individual and her own individual sleep rhythms determine her sleep requirements.

Sample routine for your preschooler

- Your preschooler may continue to wake very early, but by now she may begin to align her sleep with the family's.
- Breakfast with the family
- Going to day care
- If you're at home this will be playtime, including social time with you, toys and games
- Going for a walk in the park, riding little bikes or scooters, visiting friends
- Morning tea (usually fruit) and a drink of water
- Another playtime – play activities are always associated with her developmental age and choice. Play doesn't always have to be structured; lots of free, imaginative play is important for this age group.
- Lunch
- Another playtime
- She may have an afternoon nap of 50 minutes to 1½ hours if she's really tired.
- Afternoon tea (usually fruit) and a drink of water
- Another playtime
- Pick up from day care
- Special time with you after day care
- Dinner with the family
- Quiet, wind-down cuddle time
- A bath or shower and her bedtime routine, including reading a story together and settling for the night.

Calming bedtime routine for your preschooler

A predictable, familiar and calm bedtime routine will usually result in your preschooler falling asleep more quickly. If you've been having problems at bedtime, a calm, soothing and familiar routine may also reduce disruptive bedtime behaviours. However, your preschooler may like to extend the bedtime routine much longer than it needs to be; a bedtime routine lasting 30 to 45 minutes is enough.

Night-time routines for your preschooler usually include a bath or shower and putting on pyjamas. She may enjoy a warm milk drink, so make sure she cleans her teeth afterwards to avoid the milk remaining in her mouth and settling on her teeth. This can cause tooth decay, which means she could lose her baby teeth early and have to endure uncomfortable trips to the dentist.

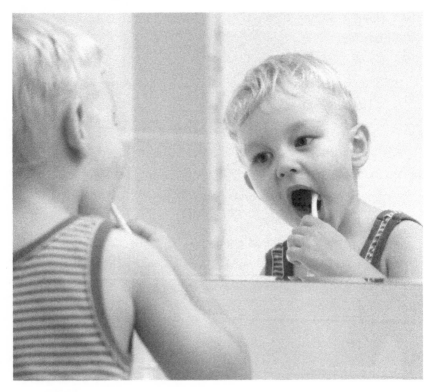

Once you've attended to teeth cleaning, you can both enjoy cuddles and a storybook or two of her choice. This is probably best done in a quiet place, such as her bed.

Avoid bright lights, lots of noise, TVs and using a smartphone or tablet. These will stimulate her and keep her awake longer.

The aim of the routine is for her to go to bed calm and relaxed enough to move into a drowsy state, ready for sleep. Once she's calm and drowsy in her bed, you give her an affectionate kiss goodnight. Just like when she was a toddler, she thrives on your affection. Her brain grows stronger and healthy neural connections are made every time you touch her gently, kiss her and tell her you love her.

If your preschooler still has a dummy or a special blanket, toy or comforter, she may want it, but by this age many children have already discarded them. During the preschool years, you have the ability to bargain with her over the dummy so she can learn to do without it – for example, she can give it to the magpies. Preschoolers like to negotiate, and why not? You like to negotiate and get something out of a bargain, don't you? If she doesn't decide to discard her dummy, you can negotiate a deal now that she's a big girl.

Remember, she may be associating the dummy as being important to her comfort. Therefore, if she's giving up something important, the deal has to worthwhile to her. You will also need to provide lots of praise and encouragement with this package deal.

The toy, blanket or comforter is more difficult. When she was a toddler, the object was chosen to provide her with comfort and security in your absence. If she still has problems going to bed or seems anxious about other things, her comfort object will remain important. She needs it to help her calm down when she gets upset.

Bit by bit, you may be able to encourage her to use her comforter only at bedtime so it becomes a bedtime association. She will decide when her comforter is no longer necessary.

Signs your preschooler may have a sleep problem

When your preschooler has a sleep problem, it impacts on both of you. You will both feel tired and exhausted, but she might not show her lack of sleep by yawning or telling you she's tired. Your preschooler will show you how tired she is through her social and emotional behaviour. Some behaviours that indicate she might not be getting enough sleep are:

- hyperactivity
- unable to control her impulses
- can't listen to you or follow your directions
- can't focus on a task
- can't take turns with friends.

Troubles with sleep

Your preschooler may have continued to have difficulties with sleep from babyhood or she may have been sleeping quite well and has suddenly begun to have troubles with sleeping.

Common sleep difficulties:

- stalling or refusing to go to bed
- trouble falling asleep
- trouble staying asleep
- TV, smartphone or tablet use prior to going to bed or using a screen in bed before sleep.

Stalling or refusing to go to bed

Your preschooler may not want to go to bed at night and will try to delay bedtime with all sorts of tactics and demands. For example, if you have a bedtime routine, she may try to extend it with requests for more stories or songs. Or she may try other ways to keep you coming to her room, such as asking for drinks, trips to the toilet, requests to watch TV with you, and she may make frequent trips from her bedroom to see you in other areas of the house.

If she continues this for 20 minutes or longer, then this is a problem. Not only is the stalling tiring for you, but she's losing sleep and will become overtired. You need to set some kind and firm limits.

> When you set a limit for your child, you're also setting limits on yourself. You have to be able to follow through.

Limit-setting for sleep

Limit-setting can be hard, especially when you're tired, but it's an important parenting skill. If you haven't done much limit-setting, start small so you and your preschooler can get used to it.

As your child grows older and develops stronger mental, social and emotional skills, limit-setting will become more important. If you can't manage to set limits for your 3-year-old, you're not going to be able set limits for your 12- or 16-year-old.

When you start with small limits and work your way up, you and your child are used to the process of making little rules and setting limits. That will make it easier for you both.

The important thing to remember about limit-setting is that, when you set a limit for your child, you're also setting limits on yourself. You have to be able to follow through and help your child with the limit you've set for both of you.

However, setting limits isn't about being stern and strict. It's a process that looks like this.

Setting limits effectively

- Provide your child with affection.
- Tell your child clearly what she has to do.
- Accept that this new limit will be hard for both of you.
- Resist your child's protests with patience and understanding.
- Resist your need to give in to her protests.
- Tell yourself you're not a bad parent.
- Tell yourself your child is not naughty.
- Praise your child for success.
- Praise yourself for success.
- Don't worry if it sometimes doesn't work, just keep trying.

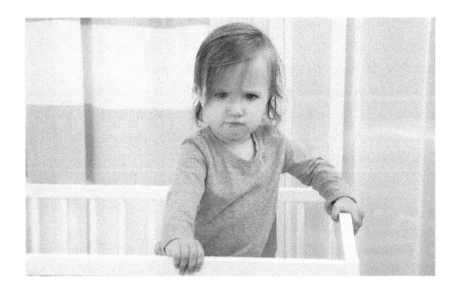

Here are some examples of things to try with bedtime stalling or when your preschooler refuses to go to bed.

Stragegies for handling bedtime stalling

- Explain to your child that she has to stay in bed and go to sleep. Also explain that you are going to help her (see the suggested settling strategies on page 220).
- Have a consistent bedtime.
- Remain firm and keep her bedtime routine to only 30 to 45 minutes.
- As part of her bedtime routine, use three to four soothing bedtime activities to help her calm down and relax.
- Resist her requests for more stories and drinks.
- Use positive reinforcement strategies, such as sticker charts and rewards, after a period of successful nights going to bed without refusing or stalling.

Trouble falling asleep and staying asleep

As your child gets older and more sociable, she will become much more interested in family goings-on. She will be especially interested in the activities of her older brothers and sisters and will want to join in with whatever they're doing. If she goes to day care, evenings can often be chaotic; she will be desperate to spend time with you and everyone is tired at the end of the day.

Under these circumstances, it's easy for some habits to develop prior to sleep that can interfere with her ability to fall asleep and/or stay asleep.

These problem habits may include:

- stimulating activities near bedtime, such as lots of rough-and-tumble games, tickling and chasing
- using her bed for activities not related to sleeping, such as playing games, watching TV or playing with electronic tablets
- consuming caffeinated drinks or foods near bedtime
- too much napping during the day
- an inconsistent bedtime.

Of course, when you look at this list of problem habits, it's not hard to see why your preschooler would have trouble falling asleep or why she keeps waking up during the night. Sometimes, it's just that you're so busy and often tired that you don't realise a normal, everyday thing could cause so much difficulty.

The main thing to do is to identify if your preschooler has any of these habits and to think about whether they could be interfering with her sleep.

Stimulating activities. These are great fun and your preschooler is probably full of beans at the end of the day. If she's been to day care, then she'll need to have some catch-up time with you to tell you about her day, just as you like to do after you get home from work.

After your reunion (she's been separated from you all day) and the catch-up time she really needs, make sure she has a good wind-down period. This can include a relaxing bath or shower and then her bedtime routine. Remember, bedtime routines need to be only 30 to 45 minutes.

Playing in bed. Make sure she understands that her bed is for sleeping only. If you think about it, playing is her daily business and her toys are the tools she uses. You don't need work-related equipment in your bed, your place for resting, and neither does she. That would be too stimulating and she needs to understand that her bed is for sleeping.

Caffeine. Pretty much everyone knows that caffeine keeps you awake, but you may not know that you're giving your child a food or drink that contains caffeine. It's best to check the ingredients label of all the types of drinks and snacks you buy to see if they contain caffeine. Unfortunately, products don't always specify caffeine, so you may wish to search the internet for sites that provide food label ingredient names for caffeine.

Foods that contain caffeine include:

- coffee, including coffee extracts and green coffee
- green, black, white and oolong teas
- kombucha (a fermented tea)
- milk chocolate, dark chocolate and cocoa in any food, including ice creams, puddings, cakes and cereals
- cola-flavoured drinks
- energy drinks
- guarana.

Too much napping during the day. Your preschooler needs only 10 to 12 hours of sleep in each 24-hour period, and she will usually have that sleep during the night. By 4 years of age, she probably won't need a daytime nap at all. But if she does have a nap, she may reduce her hours of night-time sleep.

One important question is whether or not preschoolers should have a nap at day care. There is no right or wrong answer. If your preschooler takes a nap at day care, she will probably stay up later in the evening. The answer about whether to have a nap during the day really depends on what works best for you and your preschooler.

Inconsistent bedtime. It's important to keep your preschooler to a consistent bedtime and bedtime routine because when she knows she goes to bed at a certain time, she can prepare herself. Bedtime is predictable for her and more relaxing. This set pattern also promotes the beginning of good sleep and helps her stay asleep throughout the night.

When she doesn't know what time she's going to bed and bedtime is unpredictable, then she'll play and keep busy. This may make her more stimulated later into the evening and she will find it harder to wind down.

Then, when you decide she should go to bed, she will be more likely to argue and bargain with you. She may stall and refuse to go to bed, and have trouble getting to sleep and staying asleep. This is what makes her sleep deprived and she will show that through the disruptive behaviours we looked at on page 212.

TVs, video games, computers, tablets and smartphones

Electronic devices are being used much more frequently as part of bedtime routines. You might be thinking, 'What's wrong with that? I can read stories, play games or watch movies with my child on them. We're together.' And you're right, you are together. Unfortunately, though, these devices end up replacing more soothing bedtime routines.

There are problems with viewing these screens at your preschooler's bedtime. Firstly, they have blue lights, which are very stimulating and delay melatonin production; remember, melatonin induces sleep (see Chapter 1: How sleep works). Plus, they are exciting and so much more stimulating than a real book with paper pages to turn.

Research has shown that evening screen-time use is particularly associated with sleep problems, especially if your preschooler has a TV in her room. She will go to sleep later and her sleep quality will reduce with the more hours of TV use she has. She will wake up tired and may also start to display overtired behaviours.

The other difficulty with having a TV in the bedroom is that its use is usually unsupervised once your child goes to bed. Your preschooler may be exposed to violent content, which is also known to cause sleep problems. This may cause nightmares, sleep terrors and sleep talking.

TV and screen time can also cause your preschooler to stall or refuse to go to bed and have trouble falling asleep and staying asleep. It's important to consider that any screen time she has before bed will disrupt her sleep, even if you watch TV or use the other devices with her.

If using screen time is part of your child's bedtime routine, it might be worthwhile experimenting to see if her sleep improves if you introduce a new soothing bedtime routine to replace the screen time, and keep screen time to daytime use only.

As we saw in Chapter 1: How sleep works, there's lots of research being done on the effects of blue light and screen time on babies and children, so it's important to think about how you can help your preschooler to go to sleep and sleep well through the night. At the moment, experts believe that when your child is between 2 and 5 years old, she shouldn't have any longer than 1 hour of screen time a day. When she does have her screen time, she needs to enjoy it with you as a social occasion. And, like all social occasions at this age, screen time needs to be in the morning or afternoon, well away from her bedtime so she isn't affected by the glare of the blue lights prior to settling to sleep for the night.

Reducing screen time to the recommended levels can be hard for everyone, not just for your child. It's so easy to turn on the TV for your little one or let her play a game on a tablet or game console while you do some work, so it's unfortunate that blue light and screen time have been proven to disrupt sleep.

But if you can do the amazing and reduce her screen time, once everyone's over their blue screen withdrawals, you may find some fun, creative things to do that you like more – just maybe.

When your preschooler won't settle

You've tucked your toddler into her bed but she continues to call for you or gets up to find you try these strategies to settle her for the night.

Strategies for settling your preschooler

- Gently and firmly lead her back to her own bed. Tuck her in again, kiss her goodnight and tell her it's time for sleep. You will probably have to walk her back to bed several times. Try to stay calm.
- If she gets distressed, cuddle her until she's calm and then leave the room again.
- Speak gently and quietly to reassure her, telling her, 'It's time for sleep'. Encourage a state of calm and reassurance.
- If she still doesn't respond, you could try giving her a small drink of water but nothing else.
- If she's very upset then try staying in the room until she falls asleep on her own. You could sit on a chair quietly or lie on a mattress. Don't speak to her except to gently say, 'It's time for sleep now', if she wants to keep talking.
- If she will only sleep if you stay in the room, tell her you're going to start moving your chair or mattress a little distance away each night while reassuring her you're still close by.
- As she becomes more reassured, watch to see when she becomes comfortable and less anxious about bedtime and being left to go to sleep on her own. When you see she seems ready, it's time to move out of the room.
- The length of time it takes to move completely out of the room will depend on how anxious she is about sleeping on her own.

Other aspects of sleep

There are some other aspects of your preschooler's sleep environment for you to think about if she's having sleep problems.

The temperature in her bedroom

Make sure her bedroom is a comfortable temperature for the time of year, neither too hot nor too cold. You know yourself how badly you sleep in really hot weather, and being too cold at night also affects sleep. There are no specific recommended room temperatures for children for winter or summer, but ensure that your preschooler is dressed for the weather and her bedding is warm or cool enough.

The amount of light in her bedroom

Make sure the lights in her room aren't too bright. If your child needs a night-light, ensure it casts a red or yellow light rather than a blue light (see Chapter 1: How sleep works). Exposing your child to bright lights, especially fluorescent lights, TVs, computer screens, tablets and phones, will stimulate her and keep her awake.

No loud noises to disturb her

No one can sleep if there's too much loud noise going on in the house. Loud noises are far too stimulating as well. Normal household conversations, TV volume at a low level and standard household goings-on are all perfectly okay. Your preschooler will adjust to those noises and they won't bother her at all once she's asleep.

Sleep problems can affect your preschooler in many ways. A lack of sleep will affect her ability to socialise and play with her friends, and it can also affect her mood and behaviour, causing her to be impulsive and hyperactive. Sleep problems can affect her ability to learn, listen, remember and follow rules. A lack of sleep can also affect her health and, sometimes, can lead to diagnosis of behavioural problems.

Consistency in establishing predictable sleep and daily routines throughout the day and night, and helping your preschooler learn to fall asleep on her own and sleep through the night, will reduce her sleep deprivation and daytime tiredness.

With your help, she'll sleep better, feel better and can catch up with her social and emotional development. And you'll both feel great.

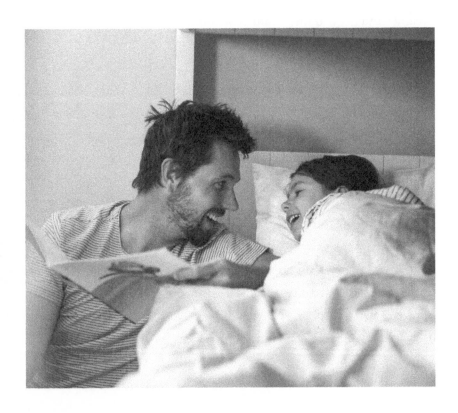

Samantha's story (mother of Naomi, 4)

Naomi was never a natural sleeper, you could say. She woke many times at night from the word go and her sleep didn't improve for years. In the beginning, I had a list of techniques that I would follow, including wrapping, patting, holding, bouncing, walking with her, driving with her. We would keep trying them all, then, as they failed, we would go to the next one. I would often be one of those mums walking around the streets at 3 am with a crying baby strapped to me. It was utterly exhausting.

After a while, we realised that noise and touch were the tools that helped the most. We would put white noise on and sing lullabies while holding her or patting her to sleep. I comforted myself with the mantra 'this too shall pass'. Babies can't possibly cry forever, so we knew we just had to hang in there and eventually she would fall asleep.

When Naomi was 3, we found out we were having a new baby, which made us think about our situation and how to change it. As the baby will be sleeping in our room, we decided that it was time for Naomi to have her own room and her own bed. I was so nervous about how it would go, but it's actually been a much easier transition than I first thought.

We brought up the idea of her own room with her and showed her the bedrooms of some of her friends. She loved the fact that they had their own spaces and wanted that for herself. So, we made a big effort to decorate her room and get her a big girl bed. We bought her a pretty doona cover and decorated the walls with images of fish and dolphins, her favourite animals.

We also introduced a reward chart – we give her a sticker for every full night she stays in her bed and when she gets five

223

stickers, she can have a treat. Sometimes it might be a small toy, sometimes we take her out for ice cream.

It took a few months for her to get used to it but these days, she's sleeping through almost every night. Sometimes she comes into our bed early in the morning but it's getting rarer and rarer. Our baby is due soon, so it was just in time!

I think she was the type of child who needed that extra attention and reassurance overnight for a bit longer than some other children. I'm really proud of her success and proud of my husband and me for getting through the sleep deprivation and coming out the other side with a happy and confident little girl.

Key message

- Your preschooler is learning to solve problems with your help and guidance, as well as stopping herself from doing something you tell her not to do. This is learning self-control, which is important for transitioning to school.
- Setting appropriate limits is a key parenting skill, but it can be hard if you haven't done much limit-setting before. If you've been having troubles with your preschooler's bedtime and sleep, you're going to need to set some limits for both of you. It's best to start small so you and your preschooler can get used to it; that way you'll be more able to stick to your new routine.
- There are two common problems that stimulate your preschooler, both of which can contribute to keeping her awake at night: consuming foods or drinks containing caffeine; and watching TV or using other electronic devices prior to bedtime, as these contain blue light, which adversely affects sleep.

CHAPTER 11

Siblings, twins, child care and sleep

This chapter will help you find answers to some common problems about how your baby's and/or child's sleep can be affected by siblings, being a twin or going to child care. First, when you add a new baby to your family, this can certainly disrupt your older child's sleep for a little while, and it's good to be prepared for that.

Having twins (or higher-order multiples) brings lots of joy and excitement, but there is much to learn about and organise with twins, and interrupted sleep is often a major factor for families with twins.

Finally, managing sleep routines between child care and home is important, and because balancing home, work, study and child care is sometimes tricky, parenting and sleep routines get a bit mixed up.

When you have two or more children, your life gets more complicated, so it's important to have realistic expectations.

A new brother or sister

You've finally got sleep figured out for your child. She's going to bed and sleeping well, often through the night. She's grown up now and in a predictable routine. Things sure are looking up and being a parent doesn't seem so hard after all. Life's sweet!

And then, something starts to happen. You start looking at other mums with their new babies and remember how delightful your little one was as a baby. Every sleepless night, if not forgotten, is forgiven. Next thing you know, you have your own delightful new baby, a welcome addition to the family. It happens to almost everyone, can't be helped. After all, babies are irresistible in spite of the lack of sleep and crying.

You believed your toddler or preschooler fully understood you had a baby in your tummy while you were pregnant. You explained she would have a new brother or sister to play with; you prepared her for the new baby, just like the books told you to do.

Your new baby finally arrives and, for a few weeks, it's all very exciting. Everything goes well for a while and then the novelty of her new baby brother wears off and your older child's behaviour starts to change. If she's a preschooler, she might be able to tell you she doesn't want that baby in the house anymore or ask you to put him back in your tummy. If she's a toddler, she may be more of a handful than usual.

If you think about it, you might be thrilled to welcome a new baby, but your toddler or preschooler wasn't part of the decision to include someone new into the family. She might not want him around. She was perfectly happy to be the only child and the centre of your attention. She didn't understand that she would have to share your time and affection.

Often, after a new baby arrives, your older child can feel replaced, angry and even rejected. These feelings are more common in first children. Make sure your older child is always included in the social events that surround a new baby. Family, friends and even strangers are drawn to babies, so the baby gets fussed over. Your toddler and preschooler may feel left out at times – and it's not nice to feel forgotten. A simple way to include her is to have her tell people the baby's name, which can prompt someone to ask for her name. All your older child needs is to be a part of the new and exciting events surrounding her new sibling.

As for you, you may feel guilty that you can't give your older child all your attention. Sometimes, it's tempting to try to keep giving her the same amount of attention as before, but now it's your new baby's turn. He needs you to give him all that love and attention you gave her when she was first born. It's vital for his brain development.

When you have two or more children, your life gets more complicated, so it's important to have realistic expectations for yourself and your little ones as you learn how to share your time with them both. You're going to be busy with the new baby, so your older child needs to actively participate in the new family routines that include the baby. An example could be she introduces 'our' new baby to friends who come to visit. Most importantly, ensure that you let her know that you still love her and show her lots of affection.

So, if you're going to give your new baby all the love and attention he needs, including the time to develop predictable routines and his day–night sleep rhythms, you might wonder how to balance that when you already have a predictable routine for your toddler or preschooler.

Balance is the key when you have two or more children – and balancing each child's needs takes practice. This is achieved by keeping both of them in mind at the same time, remembering when you do something with your new baby, to include your older child; and when you do something with your older child, to include your baby. Your older child needs to feel part of the 'team', so use phrases with her such as 'our' baby.

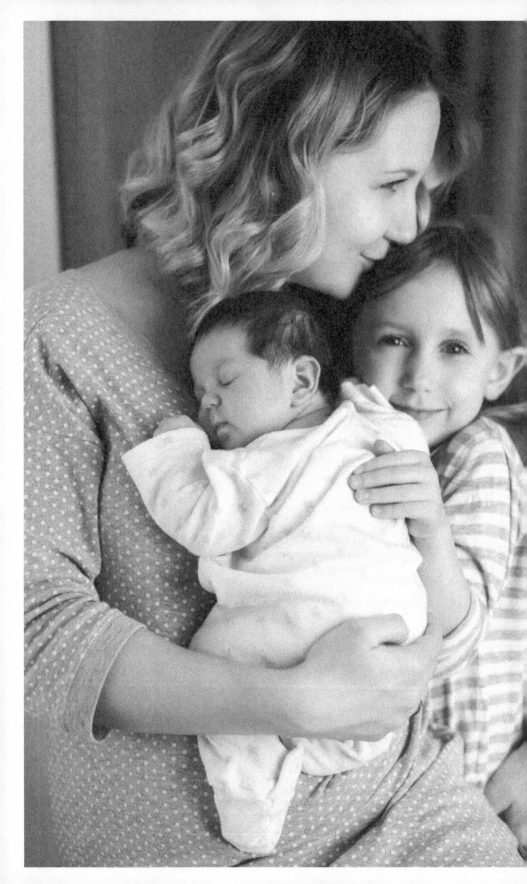

Now you're saying, 'Examples please!'

Okay, so this book is about sleeping. You're trying to establish your new baby's day–night rhythms (see Chapter 1: How sleep works), help him soothe himself to sleep and between sleep cycles (see Chapter 2: Sleeping longer through the night, and Chapter 7: Working on your sleep problems: Birth to 6 months). Your older child can't help you soothe your baby to sleep, but you can explain to her that babies need lots of sleep and what you will be doing to help your baby sleep, just like you helped her. An older sibling loves to hear about when she was a baby and how you looked after her.

Some things you can do at home to encourage her to participate or simply enjoy some time with you are:

- Explain and show her your new baby's non-verbal cues and tired signs (see Chapter 6: How your baby communicates) so she can understand his communications as well. This will help her feel more positive towards him.
- Ask her to help you prepare him for bed, bring you a nappy or his cotton wrap; or during his sleep she can listen with you for when he wakes.
- Use a doll to show her what you do when you put him to bed or settle him back to sleep. She can put her doll to bed while you settle the baby to sleep. Little boys can certainly do this as well.
- To occupy her when you have to settle the baby, bring out some special toys at baby's bedtime.
- Use some of your baby's sleep time as special time with your older child to reinforce your bond with her while doing quieter activities.

How do you include your baby when you're with your older child? That's easy. When your baby's awake, make sure he's part of social times with your older child. During the first three months, show her how he can hold her finger and smile at her. After three months, he'll be very interested in watching her play. Make sure you give him playtime with just you, as well as playtime altogether.

Establishing routines

Developing predictable routines can be tricky when you have both a new baby and a toddler or preschooler to keep entertained and engaged – you can't give up all your commitments, such as playgroups or toddler dance class. If your older child is involved in activities every day, it may be time to reassess her schedule and possibly reduce those commitments for a while. This will mean finding a compromise so that some days are free of activities. On activity-free days, you can stay at home and establish a predictable day–night sleep routine for your baby.

That might disappoint your older child, but then again it might not. She may be glad to have a break as well.

If your older child spends time at child care, it's probably a good idea to continue that routine, but make sure she has lots of reassurance. She will want to introduce 'our' baby to her friends and the teachers there.

The most important thing about having time at home is to help your baby begin life with a predictable daily routine to ensure that his sleep develops. This way, you and the rest of the family can get the good night's sleep you all need as well (see chapters 1 to 7).

As you know, if your new baby doesn't develop the ability to soothe himself to sleep and resettle between sleep cycles, everyone in the family will be sleep deprived. Give him as many of the right conditions as you can to ensure he can learn to establish his sleep rhythms.

The specific details (and memory) about establishing sleep rhythms and cycles might not have occurred to you when you dreamed about a new baby. Take heart – you've done it once and you'll be able to do it again. In fact, you may find it a little easier second time around because you have a better understanding of a baby's sleep needs and what you can do to support your new baby to develop his sleep rhythms.

On the days when you're out and about, still try to maintain a loose routine for your baby. You will recognise when he's tired and he can sleep in his pram on those days. Remember, though, it's better for him if he has a safe, familiar bed and surroundings for the majority of his sleeps.

As you might guess, shopping centres and other busy locations aren't really good places to get a restful sleep. Can you imagine what it must be like trying to sleep in a shopping centre with all those bright lights, hundreds of people and loud noises? It can be very hard for a baby to sleep there, especially while he's establishing his sleep rhythms (see chapters 1 to 3).

When you're out of the house, keep in mind that the preferred type of pram for your baby is one that faces you, so he can see your face all the time and gain constant reassurance. Imagine being in a pram at knee level and hundreds of people coming at you really fast!

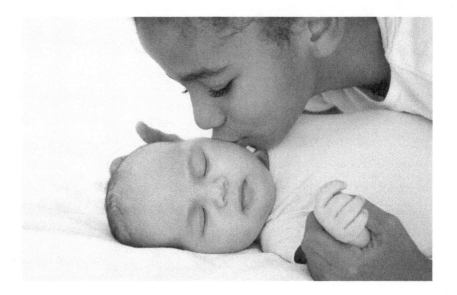

Bedtime

When you have two children, it's nice to have some help around bedtime (as well as most other times). When you are attending to the baby, your partner (or a friend or carer) can provide your older child with attention and care. The same goes for you when your partner has the baby.

It's a lot harder, of course, when you're on your own and you can't hand the baby over to someone else. Getting support from family or friends whenever you can is absolutely essential. Predictable routines are possibly even more important for you and your children when you're on your own, although sometimes they are hard to maintain.

Having a bedtime routine for both children is really important. Of course, your children will have slightly different routines, particularly during your new baby's first 12 months, and evenings can be very busy while you get them both ready for bed.

The evenings can be easier if you include your older child in actively participating in the baby's routine and make her feel important as his older sister. She can fetch and carry supplies, help bathe the baby and help dress him. Sometimes, she can even 'read' a story to him (if she's not able to read yet, she can describe her own version of familiar tales, using pictures as prompts). Once he's ready for bed, she can kiss him goodnight as she moves to another room to leave you to settle him on your own.

Make sure you maintain her consistent bedtime and regular bedtime routine, and give her plenty of love and attention at the end of her busy day. She needs her predictable routines more than ever while she negotiates so many big changes in her life. Being a big sister is tiring, and she won't always be able to tell you what she's feeling except through her behaviour (see chapters 9 and 10).

232

Handling housework

The arrival of a second baby changes so many things in family life. Finding time for both your children is often hard, let alone time for yourself, and then couple-time as well. This is a good stage to think about sorting your priorities. Housework and all the stuff that needs to be done around the house can really mess with your head because it just sits there and doesn't go away unless you give it your attention. But that's the beauty of it, right? It waits for you and doesn't care how long you take.

Your children are another matter, however. They can't wait long for your attention. The longer they wait, the more they fuss and need you.

If you really think about it, your relationship with your children and partner are the most precious things in your life. So that's where your energy needs to go. Relationships are your priority. Then you need free time to catch your breath and enjoy some moments for yourself.

After that, all that housework hanging around waiting patiently for you can be prioritised into two groups: what has to be done, and what would be nice to do. If you're totally into cleaning, prioritising and leaving something for later could be difficult for you. But then, your relationship is the most important aspect of a child's life, especially in the first three years. Decide that the cleaning can wait while you establish your new baby's day–night sleep rhythms, and while you and your two little ones all get to know each other.

Twins (and higher-order multiples) and sleep

Parenting two or more babies at once is certainly more demanding than just one baby. Developing a predictable routine for your twins is crucial. Try to coordinate the twins' feeding, socialising and sleeping routines so they are awake at the same time. If their sleeping pattern gets out of sync and one baby is deeply asleep while the other has been awake for hours, you'll be exhausted trying to manage a never-ending cycle of feeding, socialising and settling. Just as with a single baby, having predictable daily and bedtime routines is essential for twins to establish their day–night and self-soothing sleep rhythms.

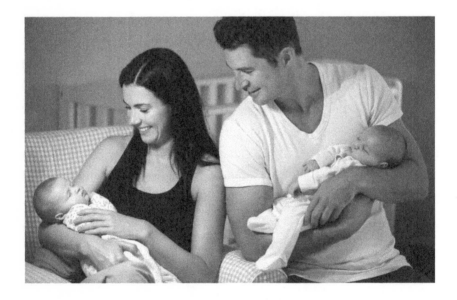

Sleeping arrangements for twins

There are differing opinions on whether you should sleep twins in the same crib or cot, called 'co-bedding', or sleep them on their own right from the start.

Studies show that about 50 per cent of parents co-bed their twins when they first get home from hospital.

You may have been told or read that co-bedding your twins from birth has advantages. Some of the advice might be: your twins may sleep better; they prefer to be together; they are easier to care for; they synchronise their breathing.

A few studies have been done to see if these beliefs hold up and some evidence has emerged to support these ideas. The best support that's been found so far is that twins do seem to synchronise their sleep states when they sleep together.

On the other hand, some parents are concerned that if their twins share a cot they may overheat, disturb each other or, in the absolute worst case, suffocate each other. The research suggests that your twins won't overheat or disturb each other. Even if one twin cries, the other twin will get used to the crying and tune it out after a while; just like you tune out the sound of regular household or outside noises while you're asleep at night.

However, it has been found that twins sleeping side-by-side can move around and occasionally cover each other's face, mouth and nose for a moment or two, which could disrupt breathing.

Tresillian follows Red Nose recommendations for the safe sleeping of your twins to reduce the risk of Sudden Unexpected Deaths in Infancy (SUDI), including SIDS.

Safe sleeping guidelines for twins

- If desired, place each twin in a separate safe sleeping bag with a fitted neck, fitted armholes (or sleeves) and without a hood; or use a firm, but not too tight, wrap with your baby's arms flexed at the chest.
- Place each twin in their own cot on their back, not on their tummy or side.
- Keep both twins in your room, in their own cot, for the first 6 to 12 months.

If you're in a temporary situation where you have only one cot, here are ways to reduce the risks when twins share one cot:
- Do not use bedding.
- If desired, place each twin in a separate safe sleeping bag with a fitted neck, fitted armholes (or sleeves) and without a hood; or use a firm, but not too tight, wrap with your baby's arms flexed at the chest.
- Place your twins on their back, not on their tummy or side, at the opposite ends of the cot, with both heads towards the middle. Do not place twins side by side.
- Babies should never co-sleep with any older children.
- When babies have reached the age when they can freely move around the cot, they must be placed in separate cots.

Synchronising routines for twins

Your twins are individuals, and by watching their non-verbal cues and tired signs and by observing their habits and preferences, you will be able to recognise the differences of when each one gets tired and how each one sleeps.

With your help, your twins may be able to partly synchronise their routines so that they are sleeping and feeding around the same times. A good way to start is to make sure your twins enjoy their day and night bedtime routines together and they are settled to sleep at the same time.

To help synchronise their sleep, try to resettle Twin A if she happens to wake between sleep cycles when Twin B remains asleep. Use this technique when you think that your twins could do with more sleep and aren't ready for a feed, so resettling is the best option for your unsettled twin. (See chapters 7 to 9 for settling techniques.)

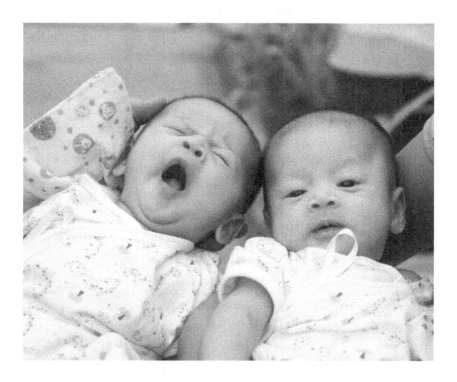

The same is also true for feed times. If Twin A wakes close to a feed but Twin B isn't awake yet, you could wait a little while before deciding to gently wake the sleeping twin (Twin B) to assist with synchronising their routine.

Remember to enjoy the times when there's just one twin awake, even if it's just for a few minutes, and make the most of this opportunity to strengthen your bond with your twins individually.

Once both twins are awake, resume their regular feeding routine, then socialise and play with them together and, hopefully, put them to sleep at the same time using their regular sleep routine.

Settling twins

So, what happens if you're having sleep and settling difficulties with your twins? Twins have exactly the same sleep and settling problems as singleton babies and with the same causes. It's a good idea to re-visit chapters 1 to 4, where we looked at how sleep develops, the two sides of sleeping problems and how important routines are.

When Twin A is unable to settle and you wish to resettle her, you can do the resettling in the same room as Twin B if it doesn't disturb him. You use the same Responsive Settling techniques described in chapters 7 to 9. However, if Twin A does disturb Twin B (and you as well) during the night, then it's okay to move Twin A to a separate room to do some Responsive Settling.

Often, one twin will not actually be disturbed by the other twin being unsettled. Try not to get too anxious about them disturbing one another; it can be surprising how many babies will sleep peacefully even when their twin wakes and cries. Observe your two individuals and get to know how they respond to these situations.

Once you've figured out what's happening between both you and Twin A and you've both resolved her sleep difficulties, Twin A can move back into your room, particularly if she's less than 6 months old.

One of the most difficult sleep issues you can experience with twins is when they synchronise their problems with settling to sleep or settling between sleep cycles. This can be very hard, so use whatever works best for you and the babies. Having the twins in the same room and in separate cots side-by-side enables you to provide some sort of rhythmic touch concurrently, such as gentle patting or stroking, while saying 'shhh, shhh' to both.

If they are keeping each other awake for too long, you could move one to a different room and settle them separately using Responsive Settling techniques (see chapters 7 to 9).

You could try attending to the calmer twin first – you may find she settles easily with a little dedicated attention, especially if it's close to the routine sleep time – and then turn your attention to settling the more unsettled twin. However, the order is up to you; you will get to know your twins best and what they need.

If both twins are very upset and crying, you could hold Twin A in your arms to soothe her and put Twin B in a rocker to calm him, rocking the chair gently with your foot. If you have a partner or carer with you, each one of you can hold and soothe a baby before trying to resettle them. For more ideas about soothing your crying baby, see Chapter 5: Why your baby cries.

Taking caring of yourself

Like all new parents experience, you will be tired. Very tired. Parents of twins need to ensure that they rest when they can. It's strange that you can be so tired, yet so wired up that resting becomes hard to achieve.

Remember to be kind to yourself and don't set overly high expectations about what you would like to achieve in a day. It can be a challenge to make yourself stop and rest when you feel overwhelmed, but if you can give yourself at least 15 minutes of rest when your babies sleep, do it. At night, go to bed when your babies go to bed.

Getting adequate rest enables you to recharge your energy levels and helps to keep your day more manageable and your emotions in check. If you're well rested and remain calm, your babies will be calmer too – well, mostly.

Try to establish and stick to coordinated, predictable daily routines for your twins. Some days, it will feel as if everything has come together like a charm, while other days may feel like chaos, with your twins taking turns to wake, feed and sleep. Just take some deep breaths, remember to enjoy the special moments looking into their eyes and tell yourself, 'I'll try again tomorrow'.

A good website to gain support and access information about parenting twins and multiples is the Australian Multiple Birth Association (amba.org.au). They have local branches throughout Australia, offering resources, education seminars, playgroups and a fantastic chance to interact with other families raising multiples.

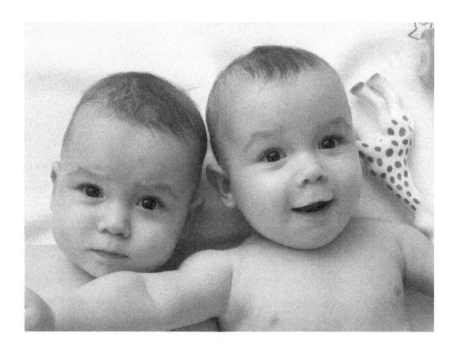

Isabelle's story (mother of 2-year-old twins, Charlotte and Angus)

Nothing can fully prepare you for the reality of life with twins. I didn't know anyone who'd had a multiple birth when I found out I was expecting twins, so it was really hard to predict just how difficult (yet rewarding) it was going to be.

I'm not going to sugar-coat it – the first year of their lives was one of the hardest years I've ever had. It started when they arrived eight weeks early and were rushed to the NICU. Although I was discharged after five days, they remained in Special Care for five weeks.

In many ways, we were lucky: they were little fighters and despite each being only a few kilos at birth, they didn't have any major health complications. The one advantage of them being in the hospital for so long was the amount of help and support we were able to get from the midwives. I was able to establish breastfeeding and learned how to twin-feed, which is a great way to save time in the early days. The midwives also helped put them into a routine, which I soon learned was essential with twins or else you won't ever sleep!

We got quite used to the hospital environment and after we left, I found being at home isolating. Leaving the house with two seemed like such a mammoth task, but I tried to do it at least once a day as it was vital to me feeling sane. I'd always give myself a good hour to prep everything I'd need to leave, to ensure I didn't get stressed. I broke everything down into little steps, like 'get the food', 'get the nappies', 'put the bag in the car', 'get Bub 1', 'put him in the car', 'get Bub 2' and so on. Each step on its own is simple but when you view it all as one giant hurdle, it makes it seem really hard.

We were shocked by how demanding and tiring it was in the early months, and although I'm a pretty independent person,

I soon learned how important it was to accept help. Whether it was home-cooked meals waiting in the freezer, our neighbours walking the dog or friends and family coming over and holding babies while we had a nap, every offer was gratefully received.

Other than our close network, I turned to a few groups for support in the early days. I joined both a regular mothers' group and a twins mothers' group. I found that I got different types of support from each and formed some amazing friendships. I also called Tresillian a lot in the early days and went to see them for a Day Stay. It's obviously pretty difficult to settle two babies at once, so we got some tips like positioning the cots so we could pat two babies at once and we got two bouncers so we could hold one and bounce the other with our feet. It's really about finding whatever works!

I've found with twins that the hardest days are in the beginning, so the older they get, the easier it gets. Now that they're 2 years old, it's just so much fun. They play together and we are learning their little unique personalities. When they run into my arms and give me a cuddle, I could just explode with happiness.

Sleep and child care

Attending a childcare centre can be stressful for your child initially because it involves a long separation from you. She loves to be with you, so any time apart creates a level of distress while she waits for you to return. A good way to help her with the separation is to prepare her in advance for this unfamiliar situation, no matter how old she is.

There is nothing wrong with taking her to child care, whether it's because you need to go to work or for any other reason, and it's normal to feel like a 'bad' parent for using child care, particularly if she cries when you leave her. Thinking you're a bad parent is nonsense, though. Your little one cries because she doesn't want to leave you. That's why you need to make sure you have 'goodbyes' when you leave her and 'hellos' when you pick her up so that she feels as comfortable and safe as possible. Over time, she will understand and be reassured that you will come back.

There are ways you can help her adjust to separating from you while she's at child care.

Remind her that tomorrow is day care or a 'school day'. Talk about her friends and remind her of her favourite carer, her favourite toys and games. As she gets older, all this will begin to make sense to her, and as she acquires more language, she'll be able to join you in the conversation.

Always remain as calm as you can in the morning. This can be hard because there's so much to do getting yourself and your little one ready, but being calm will help with the drop-off and the goodbye. As you drive to child care, stay positive, but also acknowledge she may not want to go and you know she'll miss you. Tell her you'll miss her too during the day, but you'll be back together again soon.

When you drop her off, try not to rush off. Say hello to her carer and hand her over to her 'safe' person, give her a hug and a kiss. If she's crying, clinging and desperate, you need to help her calm down. You can help by soothing and speaking gently and reassuringly; you can try distracting her with some activities or her friends. Reassure her that you'll be back later. Give her an indication of her pick-up time by selecting a certain activity, such as after her afternoon tea. Remember, she can't tell the time yet.

Once you pick her up, tell her how pleased you are to see her and give her all your attention. This reunion with you is what she's been waiting for all day. She has missed you very much and will need some time with you as soon as you get home.

This is difficult when you have so much to catch up on, but it's worth it. Half an hour or so of relaxing cuddles and talk will alleviate her stress and yours; she'll let you know when she's ready to go off and do something else. Once she's had her catch-up with you, she will probably let you get on with things without bothering you too much. She will feel relaxed, happier and will be able to sleep much better.

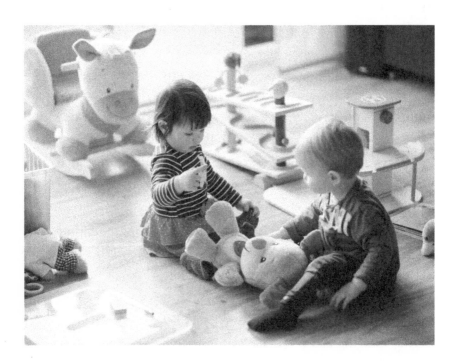

This is another moment when you need to look at her point of view. The easiest way to do that is to remember how you like to reconnect with your partner, family member or a friend at the end of your day. These catch-up times are probably after your little one has gone to bed, when you can relax and de-stress after your long day.

First of all, your little one needs a childcare centre that provides a calm and supportive environment. That doesn't mean that all the children, including yours, won't be running around and playing or the babies won't be calling out or crying. Childcare centres are busy and noisy places, but they can still have a sense of being organised, calm and supportive.

More importantly, your child needs her carers to be emotionally supportive because she will be feeling quite stressed when you leave her at the centre in the morning, especially in the early days when it is all so new and different for her. Even when she's familiar with child care and used to attending, she will still feel a certain level of stress when you leave, even if she doesn't look like she's stressed. It's normal for her to feel some stress whenever she separates from you and stays with people who aren't her special, everyday caregivers.

In the beginning of her attendance, your child will need lots of support and encouragement. Just how much will depend on her personality and temperament. She may take longer than some of the other children to settle in. If she does, it doesn't mean there's anything wrong with her, it's just that her personality and temperament make it harder for her to get used to strange places, people and longer separations from you. She needs a bit more help and encouragement.

Developing sleep routines at child care

While your child is at child care she needs to continue with her predictable daily routines and maintain naptime routines that are supportive, calm and relaxing. This is especially true for your baby, who's in the early stages of establishing her sleep rhythms and routines, and also for your toddler, who needs to maintain her predictable schedules.

> While your child is at child care she needs to continue with her predictable daily routines.

It's important that you tell her childcare educators what your child's daily and naptime routine involves and what her favourite activities are. Talk to the carers about making sure that any stimulating activities are being reduced prior to her nap time. To help her sleep, your little one needs a calm environment away from the busy play areas and a relaxing naptime routine, such as one that includes stories or cuddling soft toys.

Many childcare centres have a guideline or policy on 'sleep and rest' for the children in their care. These policies generally include sections about checking with you about your child's sleep and naptime routines. Ask if you can see their 'sleep and rest' policy so you can discuss your child's sleep needs and routine and be reassured that she won't experience too much disruption to her sleep schedule on the days she's not with you.

Your little one also needs her nap time to be free of punitive and coercive behaviour, especially if she's not ready for a nap and can't sleep. This type of behaviour probably isn't happening at your childcare centre, as most centres are well run and the childcare educators have certificate-level training or are preschool or early childhood educators. However, it's best to be alert to any changes or concerns with your child's bedtime and sleep routine behaviours that may need exploring with her childcare educators.

Another important aspect of your childcare centre to be aware of is the use of TV, laptop and tablets prior to nap time. Screen use prior to nap time is stimulating, not soothing or relaxing, so if you've already made the choice of 'no screens before sleep', make sure that her childcare educators are aware of that and support your decision.

If you have a preschooler who has stopped taking daytime naps, it's a good idea to find out what your centre's expectations are. Some centres have rest times only while other centres enable nap times for those preschoolers who still nap and offer alternative activities for those preschoolers who don't nap.

A small minority of centres still insist that every child has a nap, whether or not they need it. If your preschooler has stopped napping this could prove a problem for her, especially if the naptime period is an hour or more and she has no alternative but to lay there. In this situation she may get restless, naughty or even aggressive. When you pick her up from care, you may be told she had some behavioural problems that day, which would be very unfair. You would definitely need to discuss that situation with the childcare educators to discover what the expectations are for your little one at nap time if she can't sleep.

It's not fair to expect a preschooler to lay still and do nothing for an hour or more. She doesn't have the mental, social or emotional capacity to do that (see Chapter 10: Your preschooler and sleep). This would be a time to strongly speak up on her behalf.

By the time your preschooler is about 3 years old, she probably won't need a daytime nap on most days, although about 30 per cent of 3-year-olds still take a regular daytime nap. She now needs 10 to 12 hours of sleep in every 24-hour period, which is usually taken during the night. If she takes a 1- to 2-hour nap during the day, she will probably stay up later than usual, she may not sleep for as long or napping may disrupt her sleep at night.

If she does stay up later in the evening, you might not mind because you can both enjoy an extra hour or so together at the end of the day. For your child, having a nap at day care may not be a big deal, especially if her night-time sleep is not disrupted.

If her sleep is disrupted, however, you will need to investigate the childcare policy on preschool naps and discuss with her educators how to reduce or eliminate her naps while she's there. Instead of a nap, she could have a rest period where she engages in quiet activities. Ultimately, it should be your decision whether your preschooler has a nap at child care, nobody else's.

Sleep at preschool can be a little more difficult because the childcare educators have many children to care for and supervise. Nevertheless, it's important that you ensure your child is in a childcare centre that supports her predictable daily routines and provides a calm and emotionally supportive environment to help you maintain your child's sleep and naptime routines.

In this chapter, we looked at how different situations in your child's life affect her sleep. Having a new brother or sister can be stressful because she can feel left out or forgotten, when once she was the centre of attention. Her behaviour may change and until she develops proper language skills, she can't tell you how she's feeling.

As we have discussed, twins have the same sleeping difficulties as single babies and it's valuable to establish predictable, consistent feeding and sleeping routines. You can use the same Responsive Settling techniques (see chapters 7 to 10), with just a few modifications to enable you to settle one twin so as not to wake the other.

Going to child care is also a big event for your baby or child. While she is at child care she needs to continue with her predictable daily routines. This is especially true for your baby, who's in the early stages of establishing her sleep rhythms and routines.

Key message

- When you bring a new baby home, such an important event can affect many aspects of your older child's development, including her sleep. Be aware of how she feels with the arrival of a new baby and remember to include her in the new family relationships.
- Try to synchronise your twins' feeding, socialising and sleeping routines so they wake and sleep at nearly the same time.
- When you start to use child care, talk to your childcare provider about your little one's sleep routines so her sleep doesn't get too disrupted and you avoid sleep difficulties at home.

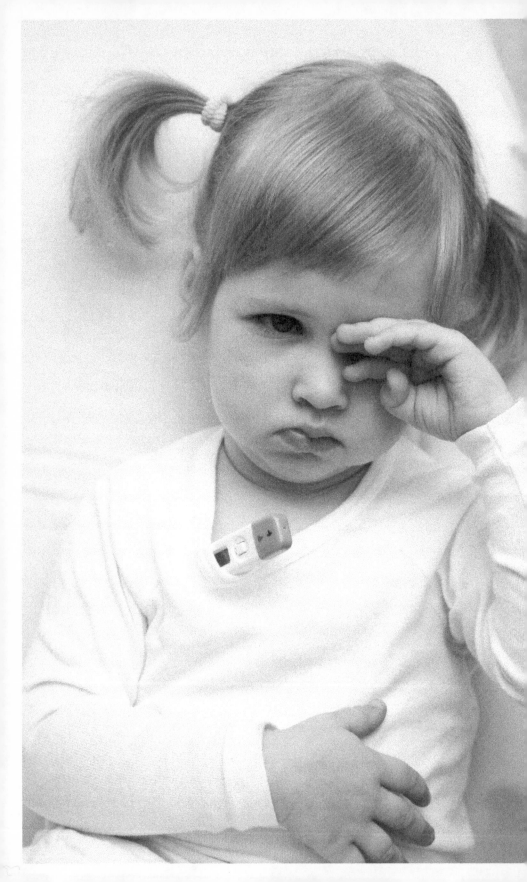

CHAPTER 12

Common illnesses and other sleep disruptions

Most children experience a range of common difficulties that affect sleep, some of which are related to a baby or child's physical health. In this chapter, we discuss the most common issues you may encounter, their symptoms, ways to treat them and what to do about your child's sleep. Here's what's covered so you can find the section relevant to you:

- infant colic
- gastro-oesophageal reflux (GOR)
- gastro-oesophageal reflux disease (GORD)
- other sleep-related problems:
  - nightmares
  - night-time fears
  - night terrors
  - head banging, body rocking, head and body rolling
- common childhood illnesses:
  - coughs
  - ear infections
  - fevers
  - the common cold

Get medical help immediately anytime your baby or child becomes unresponsive to you, if she has a fit or seizure, a fever or a rash.

251

Infant colic

If your baby has colic, she's not alone. Anywhere from 5 to 19 per cent of healthy, well-fed babies get colic, especially at around 4 to 6 weeks of age.

Everybody has an opinion on colic and they'll usually give it to you. They might say your baby has a tummy ache or wind.

But what is colic? To tell you the truth, there's still a lot of uncertainty among experts about what colic actually is and what causes it. There's debate about whether there's just one cause or multiple causes. Quite a lot of scientific studies are being done to understand why your baby might experience colic.

Of course, that bit of information doesn't help you while you're trying to calm down your extremely distressed baby each evening.

So, it doesn't really matter what's specifically causing the colic – what matters is the effect it has on you and your baby. Having a baby who cries all the time can be stressful, and your baby is experiencing a lot of distress as well. She doesn't understand what's happening to her.

One of the most difficult aspects of colic and excessive crying is that it can affect your relationship with your baby, your partner and your family. And all that crying will also affect your baby's sleep, so it's useful to understand a bit about colic.

You have probably seen your doctor, child and family health nurse or other health professional many times already for help and advice. You may have received conflicting opinions and lots of different remedies. Don't worry, you're not alone, this is a common pattern when you have a baby who cries a lot.

If you criticise yourself because you can't figure out what's wrong with your baby, well don't! You're not a bad parent; you're a confused parent.

Seeing as no one is quite sure what the cause of colic is, the best thing to do is focus on ways to manage it. If you do that, you can feel good about yourself as a parent.

During her first three months, your baby will cry between 1 to 5 hours a day, even if she doesn't have colic. That's the normal crying period for her age (see Chapter 5: Why your baby cries). Whenever your baby happens to cry at the extreme end of the crying spectrum, people may call this 'colic'.

Definition of colic

The most common expert definition of colic is called the 'rule of three', and this is how it works. Your baby is healthy and well fed and she:

1. has sudden and intense episodes of unsoothable crying and fussing for what seems like no reason at all
2. cries for more than 3 hours a day on at least 3 days a week
3. cries for more than 3 weeks.

Having said that, you're probably too caught up with all the crying to know if your baby is crying that much – for you, it just feels like she's crying all the time.

You may have been told that when your baby has colic she may also display some of these behaviours:

- her muscles seem stiff
- arches her back
- draws up her legs
- her tummy is swollen – which may be wind or she's had lots of feeds to try to calm her, so she's feeling very full
- clenches her fists
- windy and farting – this probably is more a result of crying so much rather than being the cause of the colic
- struggles when she's held.

Even if your baby doesn't have colic, you will see some of these behaviours during the first three months. These behaviours are non-verbal cues and she will show more of them if she's crying a lot (see Chapter 6: How your baby communicates). These symptoms don't necessarily mean she's in pain, even if she looks like she is.

Possible remedies for colic

So, what about all those remedies that have been suggested to you? Many remedies are based on the idea that colic has a physical cause. Not all experts agree that colic is a physical problem, that's why there are lots of different colic remedies.

Changing formula or weaning from breastmilk. If your baby has been diagnosed by your GP or paediatrician with lactose intolerance, they may suggest a change to one of the new specialised hypoallergenic formulas.

Scientific studies are uncertain on whether soy formulas are helpful for colic. If you think your baby has a cow's milk allergy, have her checked by your GP or paediatrician before changing her formula or using a specialised formula.

Importantly, if you're breastfeeding, you definitely don't have to wean her.

Excluding cow's milk from your diet during breastfeeding is rarely required, and you should seek advice from your GP or dietitian first.

Using medications. Colic usually resolves by the time your baby is 4 months old. Occasionally, it may last to 6 months, which to you will seem like forever.

There are a number of 'colic remedies' that can be purchased as over-the-counter medicine from chemists, but there is no evidence that these are effective, and some may have side effects. Tresillian does not recommend the use of over-the-counter medications for colic.

Alternative therapies. Herbal teas are thought to help with colic but there needs to be much more research done to prove this, and some can also cause serious side effects.

Chiropractic and osteopathic remedies have been studied and the evidence suggests they don't show a reduction in crying.

Massage has been shown to have some benefits. If you like to massage your baby, you can do this once a day, for one week. She might begin to relax and the length of her crying bouts may decrease.

Behavioural interventions. Make an appointment to see your paediatrician or child and family health nurse for advice on feeding, winding and burping a colicky baby.

There are a number of useful strategies for you, your partner, friends and family to try to help calm your baby. Even if she doesn't seem to like it, when she's distressed what she needs most of all is close human contact. You are her favourite person and she will be reassured by you soothing and calming her. However, you can't possibly manage her crying all the time, so when you need a break, someone else she's familiar with can take her and provide any of these strategies for her.

When she's really distressed she needs soothing touch, a soft and calming voice, gentle movements and containment and safety. That's usually in your arms or swaddled in a soft cotton wrap.

Calming techniques for colic

- rocking gently
- carrying her in a pouch
- playing soft music or white noise
- going for a walk in the pram
- giving her a warm bath
- singing lullabies and other songs softly.

Colic affects your baby's sleep. Take the time to read back over chapters 1 to 4 to review the first three months of your baby's life, how her sleep develops and the importance of predictable routines; Chapter 7 for sleep and settling, birth to 6 months; and Chapter 5 for how to manage crying.

Ensuring you get support from your family and friends is vital. You can't look after a very unsettled baby who cries 4 or more hours a day on your own. No one should expect you to do that. That's not a good idea for either you or your baby because you won't enjoy being with each other. Having a baby isn't meant to be like that, so you need someone to help you get your confidence back and get you through the 3 to 4 months that colic and crying usually last.

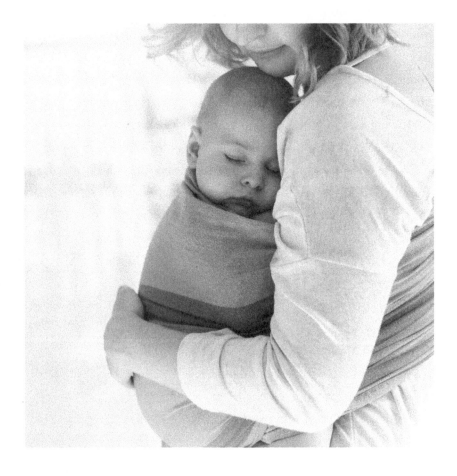

GOR and GORD: two types of reflux

Gastro-oesophageal reflux (GOR) is a common occurrence in many healthy, well-fed babies. It is physical condition. Your baby has a circle of muscle at the top of her tummy that's supposed to stay closed and keep the milk down. If she has GOR, this muscle relaxes and allows milk to come back out. About 40 per cent of babies have GOR and it usually starts before your baby is 8 weeks old.

Your baby can bring up some milk after or between feeds as many as six times a day. Other times, she may simply spill a little bit of milk from her mouth. As she gets older, however, the reflux will decrease and, by the time she's 12 months old, it will usually be gone altogether.

> Your baby can bring up some milk after or between feeds as many as six times a day.

Some babies can continue to have GOR through the first year, but it usually doesn't hurt or bother them. Take heart, only 5 per cent of babies still have GOR at 12 months, so it's not very common to continue past that point. GOR usually resolves itself and disappears as your baby matures. Even though she brings up some milk, most babies will continue to feed well and gain weight.

You may have noticed that when your baby does bring up her milk, she does it without any effort. Many babies are not distressed by this at all because it's simply the contents of her tummy coming back up into her oesophagus and into her mouth. If she's not distressed, is putting on weight and doesn't show any signs of pain, then she really doesn't need any treatment or medicine.

The milk she brings up usually isn't much, although it might look like it. Sometimes you might worry that she's brought up a whole feed. With GOR, the amounts your baby typically brings up are quite small, with the occasional large vomit if her tummy is over full.

Estimating amount of milk that comes up

A good way to get a sense of the amount she's bringing up is to tip 20 ml of water onto a cloth, let it soak in (it usually spreads quite a long way) and then compare that area to the amount of milk your baby has brought up.

GOR is normal for some babies, so if your baby has GOR then it probably won't change the amount of crying she does during the first three to four months. It just so happens that GOR usually occurs at the same time as her peak crying period; therefore, it may seem as if the GOR is causing her to cry with pain and you may be worried something is wrong with your baby. That's an easy mistake to make. (It's a bit like colic appearing around the same time.)

The main problem with GOR is that it's messy. You spend a lot of time cleaning up. If your baby tends to bring up a lot of milk, you might wear regurgitated milk stylishly on your shoulder or as a badge of endurance on the front of your clothes. You will belong to the bib-brigade you promised yourself you would never join. The only solution is to choose fashionable bibs to get you through this phase.

Gastro-oesophageal reflux disease (GORD) is much less common than most people think. Simple GOR is frequently mistaken for the more serious GORD, which leads to more severe symptoms that need assessment by your doctor and possibly medical treatment.

Symptoms of GORD

These are the symptoms of GORD to look out for:

- frequent vomiting
- she brings up large amounts of milk when she vomits
- refusal to feed
- poor weight gain and failure to thrive
- she may have a persistent cough but no sign of a cold.

Excessive crying and behaviours such as back arching and irritability aren't symptoms of GORD. Your baby will be going through a period of increased crying at the same time as the appearance of this, similarly to colic and GOR. She will often be crying and distressed during this period anyway. The difference is, she may have GORD if she also has the symptoms listed above.

Treatment for GORD requires a visit to your GP or paediatrician to investigate the reason for the frequent vomiting and large amounts of milk that comes up, as well as the other symptoms. Importantly, you do not have to discontinue breastfeeding if your baby has GORD.

Medications aren't always required as the first treatment, and they should be used only when other methods have proved unsuccessful.

These are some methods that can be tried first:

- keeping your baby upright after feeding
- asking your doctor or child and family health nurse about thickening her feeds
- giving her antacids at the direction of your doctor.

She will be very unhappy and uncomfortable at times. Imagine vomiting all the time and probably having heartburn. She probably won't find it easy to go to sleep and you will have to cope with the distress both you and she are feeling. Getting support from your family, friends, doctor and child and family health nurse is essential.

Other sleep-related problems

Sleep-related problems are common during the first three years. About 20 to 30 per cent of children experience:

- nightmares
- night-time fears
- night terrors
- head banging, body rocking, head and body rolling.

Some problems are more common than others, but most healthy and normally developing children will experience one or more at some point throughout childhood. Some of these sleep problems can make you feel really worried and concerned, but all of them usually resolve as your child matures and grows up.

Nightmares

Nightmares are vivid, terrifying dreams that occur during active sleep. Generally, your child will wake up and call for you when she has one. She will wake quickly, so the management is to comfort and soothe her. She will usually respond straightaway to reassurance that you're with her and the nightmare isn't real. But you may have to stay with her for a while if she is scared to return to sleep.

Bad dreams are different to nightmares: even though bad dreams can be scary, they don't usually wake your child up and are much more common than nightmares.

Nightmares usually occur in the second half of the night and it's thought that the onset of nightmares occurs when your child has the language development to tell you what the nightmare was about. Your preschooler generally has nightmares about threats to her safety – that's why she dreams about monsters, scary creatures or people.

Nightmares are common and it's thought that almost all children will have at least one nightmare during their early years. However, the occurrence of regular nightmares is relatively rare, with only about 1 to 4 per cent of children experiencing them frequently.

Nightmares are common and it's thought that almost all children will have at least one nightmare during their early years.

If your child is having frequent nightmares, it's usually due to some sort of stress, such as family conflict, social exclusion by children or bullying from another child at preschool. The resulting stress experienced by your child can result in her having nightmares.

If your family is experiencing a period of conflict, parental anxiety or separations, then it's important to understand the social and emotional impact on your little one. Nightmares, night-time fears and behavioural problems during the day are some of the ways she'll tell you she's not coping. This is the time to get some support for you and the family.

If there are no family difficulties and she goes to day care or preschool, investigate if there's a problem with another child or even an educator. This is a matter of discussing with the educators and making sure your child feels safe and secure.

Night-time fears

It's pretty normal for preschoolers to have night-time fears. Almost all children will at some time or other express fear of the dark, scary dreams or monsters, but with your help these fears usually disappear by 5 to 6 years of age. However, some night-time fears can be associated with heightened anxiety due to separation from you, family conflicts, parental anxiety, or your child may be experiencing trouble at preschool.

The management of night-time fears varies with the cause and the severity of her fear.

Managing fears about darkness and monsters

- If your child is very fearful of the dark, you can try putting a night-light in her room or soft lighting outside her bedroom.
- You can find a bedtime story that discusses fear of the dark and monsters under the bed or in cupboards to help reassure her they are not real.
- Try not to reinforce the idea that there could be a monster. For example, don't go searching for monsters in every nook and cranny every night before she goes to bed. If your child is very fearful, this behaviour could reinforce that there are monsters somewhere in the house. Explain to her there are no monsters and they are imaginary.
- Gently reassure her that you would never let anything bad happen to her.
- Encourage her to talk and think of what makes her bedroom and her bed a nice place to be. Most 4-year-olds are usually pretty good at describing positive aspects. Thinking about pleasant things is much better than monsters or worrying.
- Talk about how brave she is and reward her for her bravery – this could be in the form of a star chart.
- She might like to have a special stuffed animal or toy that's soothing and comforting.

The management of night-time fears related to your child's anxiety because of family difficulties, parental anxiety and preschool conflicts is a bit more challenging, especially if you are going through a difficult period in your life.

Managing anxieties about personal situations

- Use the strategies listed earlier, leaving out any advice that applies to fear of monsters and the dark.
- Find stories to read to her about children in similar situations.
- Help her to relax with a soothing bedtime routine.
- Sometimes your child will use bedtime stalling (see page 213) to express her anxiety about the family situation. You can use the techniques on page 215 to help her stay in bed
- You need to give her reassurance, understanding and support during the period of family upheaval. Your child will be emotionally affected by family conflict no matter how young she is and this will affect her sleep.

Night terrors

Night terrors usually occur between 2 to 4 years of age, although sometimes toddlers as young as 18 months can have them. After this, night terrors begin to resolve, and only 1 to 6 per cent of children between the ages of 4 and 12 years will continue to have them.

Night terrors occur when your child is in a deep sleep or quiet sleep state during the first half of the night.

Indicators of night terrors

Initially, your child will scream and when you go to her, she may display some of the following behaviours:

- look terrified with her eyes wide open
- be trembling and sweating
- be sitting up
- push you away
- get more upset when you attempt to comfort her
- seem confused and not recognise you
- wake briefly and be confused and disoriented.

This episode could last for 30 seconds to a few minutes and will then just settle on its own. Once it's over, your child usually settles back to sleep.

She probably won't remember the night terror or, if she does, it will be fragments of scary things. As for you, you'll find it very frightening the first time it happens.

Managing night terrors

- Maintain a predictable and soothing bedtime routine.
- Eliminate screen time, scary stories, movies and games.
- Eliminate drinks that contain caffeine to ensure that your child's sleep is not interrupted and decreased in length.
- Ensure she has a reasonable bedtime for her age, to avoid her becoming sleep deprived.
- Don't wake her up or restrain her, as this may prolong the episode.
- If she doesn't remember the episode, don't tell her about it, as this may just make her feel anxious.

Night terrors occur in a small percentage of children and they usually disappear during childhood. The good thing about them is your child won't remember having a night terror, so you are the one who experiences the alarm when an episode occurs. Be reassured that a night terror every so often is not a cause for concern.

Head banging, rocking, body and head rolling side to side

These sleep problems are self-soothing behaviours your child uses to get to sleep. They involve rhythmic and repetitive body movements when she's falling asleep or at any stage during sleep.

If your child does any of these sleep behaviours, she will probably start around 6 to 9 months. This may happen even when she is quite healthy and growing normally. She will usually outgrow such behaviour in early childhood. Most children don't hurt or damage themselves when they do this, though sometimes your child may bruise her forehead or develop a forehead callous. In this case, you will probably need to visit your doctor just for a check-up. There aren't any specific treatments for this particular sleep problem but here are some simple safety measures to implement.

Safety measures for head banging, rocking and rolling

- Make sure that her cot is well made and won't rock and move. Make sure it can withstand her constant rocking movements. Check all the screws are tight.
- Protect your child from falls by always keeping the cot sides up or, if your child is in a bed, use bed rails, or she can sleep on a mattress on the floor.
- Make sure she can't hurt herself on a hard object like a wall, shelf or other furniture. Move her bed away from anything she can hurt herself on.
- See your doctor if you think your child is harming herself.
- Don't use padding or bumpers in her cot to protect her head, as this is not recommended by Red Nose. Check their website (rednose.com.au) for information about bumpers and pillows.

Researchers have suggested behavioural strategies you can try. Continue to use safety measures (above) and include the following rhythmic behaviours for her self-soothing head banging or rocking.

Soothing strategies for head banging, rocking and rolling

1. Replace her rhythmic movement with your own soothing rhythmic touch, such as gentle, rhythmic patting or stroking. Keep rhythmically soothing until she's calm and sleepy.
2. Once she's soothing with your help, slowly reduce your patting or stroking and introduce a rhythmic sound, such as repetitive white noise or a fun clock with loud ticking. There are lots of children's bedroom clocks to choose from.
3. It may not happen quickly, but you should be able to stop patting or stroking completely after a period of time.

Common childhood illnesses

As if getting your child to sleep through the night wasn't hard enough, you have to contend with common childhood illnesses interfering with sleep. Colds, fevers and a bad cough all cause disruptions to sleep routines.

When your baby gets sick, her sleep will be disrupted in the short term. Once she's better, you can return to business as usual and get her back into her routine. However, take a moment to look at it from her point of view. If she's been having lots of cuddles and attention through the night, she's not going to give that up easily. She's not being naughty; she's just being like anyone else who has to give up something special. That's being human.

In the meantime, if you do have trouble convincing her to return to her previous sleep routine, check through the earlier chapters for the appropriate settling strategies for her age.

The common cold

Your child can have 6 to 12 colds every year. She experiences the common cold just like you do. Her symptoms will be a blocked and runny nose, headache, watery eyes, a cough, sore throat, mild fever and, just like you, she will feel absolutely miserable.

Colds are usually caused by viruses, so antibiotics won't be any help. And there's no specific treatment that will make a cold go away. It's a matter of waiting it out over 7 to 10 days.

In the meantime, any treatment for your baby or child will involve lots of cuddling, sympathy and attention from you. She will be clingy and probably won't sleep well.

Apart from that you can try the usual remedies. As you know from your own experience, a blocked nose is probably the worst part of a cold. Your baby's nasal passages are so small she will be very uncomfortable and will find feeding and sleeping difficult.

Ensure she has plenty of fluids, and keep breastfeeding or bottle-feeding as normal.

You can use saline sprays or nasal drops for 2 to 3 days to help clear her nose, but it's important to speak to the pharmacist to make sure you're using the right medicines for her age.

Ensure she has plenty of fluids, and keep breastfeeding or bottle-feeding as normal. If your older child isn't hungry, that's fine so long as she drinks plenty of fluids.

If your baby or child has a fever of 38.5°C or higher, you can try to lower her fever using liquid paracetamol or ibuprofen. Carefully follow the instructions on the medication label, make sure you have the correct paracetamol or ibuprofen for her age and use the recommended dosage and frequency. Don't give your child paracetamol or ibuprofen for more than 48 hours without seeing your doctor. If she has a persistent fever or you are concerned about your child's health, see your doctor for a check-up and advice.

Decongestants and cough medicines aren't recommended for children under 6 years of age. If you think your child needs some other type of medicine, then it's best to visit your doctor.

Coughs

Coughing is a symptom of an illness and it usually accompanies a cold, fever or even an ear infection. Usually, a cough will go away on its own. If your child has a persistent cough, it is best to have this checked by your doctor.

Coughs can also be caused by the exposure of your little ones to household irritants, such as cleaning sprays, disinfectants and cigarette smoke. These can irritate your child's airways and cause her to cough. Make sure that anyone who smokes goes outside the house; be mindful that cigarette smoke also stays on hands, clothes and furnishings.

Croup. Croup is another reason why your child may have a cough. Caused by a viral infection, croup can occur in children usually aged between 6 months and 3 years, and it occurs mostly at night.

Symptoms of croup

- barking cough
- wheezing
- gasping sound as she breathes
- looks as if she's working hard to breathe
- may have a fever
- may seem okay even though she's coughing.

If your child has croup, try not to panic as this will just distress her even more. Hold her calmly in a position she's comfortable in and see a doctor for treatment.

Fevers

Your child has a fever when her temperature is 38°C or higher. A fever is a sign she has an illness and is fighting an infection of some sort. Most childhood illnesses are caused by viruses, which don't need antibiotics and last only a few days.

Symptoms of a fever

- feels hot and dry
- is irritable
- may be sleepy or lack of energy
- may cry, fuss and be very clingy
- vomits or seems very unwell
- has a lack of appetite
- may shiver when her fever is rising and sweat when her fever falls.

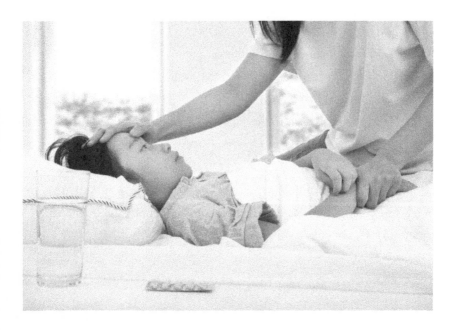

Treating a fever

What you can do when your baby or child has a fever:

- If you're concerned about her, see your doctor.
- Make sure she has plenty of fluids.
- Make sure she has lots of rest.
- Dress her in enough clothes so she doesn't shiver.
- Babies under 6 months need extra breastfeeds to avoid dehydration. If your baby takes formula, you can try some extra formula or cooled boiled water.
- If your baby or child has a fever of 38.5°C or higher, you can try to lower her fever using liquid paracetamol or ibuprofen. Carefully follow the instructions on the medication label, make sure you have the correct paracetamol or ibuprofen for her age and use the recommended dosage and frequency. Don't give your child paracetamol or ibuprofen for more than 48 hours without seeing your doctor.
- If your baby is under 3 months of age and has a fever of 38°C, take her to see the doctor straight away.
- Watch carefully to see if your child's illness is getting worse and if you think it is, go straight to your doctor or emergency room.
- Importantly, note that it is not recommended to give her a sponge bath with warm water or blow a fan on her.

Ear infections

Ear infections are common in the first six to 18 months. This is because your baby's ear canals are small and can become blocked easily. Ear infections mostly involve the middle ear and usually occur when your child has a common cold. Ear infections cause your child a lot of pain.

Symptoms of an ear infection

- clinginess
- pulling at her ears or pushing her fingers into her ears
- irritable, cranky or crying
- it might seem that she's being naughty, but she's not; she just can't tell you how much her ears are hurting
- a yellow discharge coming from her ears
- cold symptoms, such as a blocked or runny nose
- fever.

Treating ear infections

- If you think your baby or child is in pain or has a fever of 38.5°C or higher, you can try to lower her fever using liquid paracetamol or ibuprofen. Carefully follow the instructions on the medication label, make sure you have the correct paracetamol or ibuprofen for her age and use the recommended dosage and frequency. Don't give your child paracetamol or ibuprofen for more than 48 hours without seeing your doctor.
- If the ear infection is a viral illness, it should clear up after a few days without the need for any antibiotics.
- If your baby or child doesn't seem to get better, take her to see your doctor to check if her ear infection needs treatment.

All of these common problems and illnesses will disrupt your little one's daily naps and night-time sleep. You can't avoid the disturbance to her daily routine and bedtime routine. She will want all your attention most of the day and be really clingy.

If you go to work, you may have to stay home to look after your little one, as day-care centres won't allow you to bring your child in when she's sick. She will need to miss a day or two until she's better. That can be difficult for you as you juggle your work and other commitments and may have a financial impact if you don't have sick leave or carer's leave.

With your worries, it can be hard to focus, but your baby will need you to look at it from her point of view. She hasn't experienced common colds, ear infections, fevers, coughs, croup, colic or reflux before (or even if she has), and not only will she be uncomfortable but she can also be distressed and scared – that's why she's clingy. She's saying to you, 'I don't like this. I don't understand what's happening to me. Help me with this new and uncomfortable experience.'

She needs you to be calm and reassuring when she asks to be held; that's what she needs from you to get her through her first encounters with the awful common cold or colic. And you know that the more cuddling and reassuring you do when she's little, the more confident she'll be as she grows up, and she'll cope better with colds and other common illnesses she gets along the way.

As for her sleep, it will be disrupted. But once she's better again you can return to your predictable yet flexible routines and use the soothing and settling strategies suitable for her age.

Key message

- If your baby has colic, swaddle her and carry, cuddle, rock and speak to her in a calm, soothing voice.
- If your child has night-time fears, ask her to think about all the nice things about her bedroom and how safe it is, as well as telling her you'll always keep her safe.
- If your baby has a temperature of 38.5°C or higher, you can try to lower her fever using liquid paracetamol or ibuprofen. Carefully follow the instructions on the medication label, make sure you have the correct paracetamol or ibuprofen for her age and use the recommended dosage and frequency. Don't give your child paracetamol or ibuprofen for more than 48 hours without seeing your doctor.
- Importantly, note that a giving her a sponge bath or using a cooling fan for a fever is no longer recommended.

Help and where to find it

This book is a guide to help you understand your baby's normal sleep development and learn how to help her sleep development along. However, it's only a guide, and like many of the mums and their babies in the vignettes throughout this book, sometimes your situation can feel out of control.

This section will provide you with a list of services in your state or territory where you can find help for parenting your baby. It will also direct you to websites that present the latest evidence on your baby's early brain development and the importance of your baby's social and emotional development.

Emergency numbers

For serious illness or injury, call 000

For poison emergency in Australia, call 13 11 26

NSW Poisons Information Centre, also covers ACT residents: poisonsinfo.nsw.gov.au/

Victorian Poisons Information Centre: austin.org.au/poisons

Queensland Poisons Information Centre: childrens.health.qld.gov.au/ chq/our-services/queensland-poisons-information-centre/

Family care centres

All family care centres require a referral from a child and family health nurse, GP or other health professional. Some residential services may also request that you attend a local community-based day service prior to residential admission. For information about your nearest day service or residential program, and other extensive services on offer, visit the websites that follow.

Tresillian Family Care Centres (NSW & VIC)

Seven centres in New South Wales and Victoria. Day services in Wollstonecraft, Nepean, Canterbury, Lismore, Wagga Wagga (Murrumbidgee) and Albury-Wodonga. Residential services in Willoughby, Nepean and Canterbury.

Website: tresillian.org.au

Tresillian Live Advice: johnsonsbaby.com.au/tresilian_registration (Mon–Fri, 5 pm to 11 pm)

Parent Helpline: 1300 272 736 (Mon–Sun, 7 am to 11 pm)

Karitane (NSW)

Day services, plus two residential services:
Carramar and Camden

Website: karitane.com.au

Karitane Careline: 1300 227 464 (Mon–Thurs, 12:30 pm to 9 pm and 11 pm to 6 am; Fri–Sat, 9 am to 3:30 pm; Sun closed)

Queen Elizabeth II Family Centre (ACT)

Residential service in Curtin, Canberra

Website: cmsinc.org.au

O'Connell Family Centre (VIC)

Residential and day-stay service in Canterbury, Melbourne

Website: health-services.mercyhealth.com.au/our-locations/
oconnell-family-centre

QEC – Queen Elizabeth Centre (VIC)

Residential and day-stay service in Noble Park, Melbourne

Website: qec.org.au

Tweddle (VIC)

Residential service in Footscray, Melbourne, and six day-stay services:
Maribyrnong, Geelong, Bacchus Marsh, Terang, Brimbank and
Whittlesea.

Website: tweddle.org.au

Torrens House (SA)

Residential service in South Terrace, Adelaide

Website: cyh.com/SubContent.aspx?p=137

Parent Helpline: 1300 364 100 (7 days a week, 7:15 am to 9:15 pm)
Calls received outside these hours are automatically redirected
to the national Healthdirect Helpline.

Ngala (WA)

Residential and day-stay service in Kensington, Perth

Website: ngala.com.au

Ngala Parenting Line: 08 9368 9368 and 1800 111 546 –
for country callers (Mon–Sun, 8 am to 8 pm)

Ellen Barron Family Centre (QLD)
Residential service in Chermside, Brisbane
Website: childrens.health.qld.gov.au/chq/our-services/community-
health-services/ellen-barron-family-centre

Plunket (NZL)
A number of centres (or hubs) located around New Zealand. Plunket
nurses provide home and clinic visits as well as mobile clinics.
Website: plunket.org.nz
PlunketLine: 0800 933 922 (24 hours a day, 7 days a week)

Infant mental health

Australian Association for Infant Mental Health Inc. (AAIMHI)
Highlights the importance of the healthy social and emotional
development of babies and children from birth to 3 years of age. AAIMHI
has important guidelines on controlled crying and using time out.
Website: aaimhi.org/key-issues/position-statements-and-guidelines

Zero to Three
Focuses on the importance of the first three years of life and
how critical relationships are to the healthy social and emotional
development of babies and children.
Website: zerotothree.org

Center on the Developing Child, Harvard University
Presents easy-to-understand research about the critical importance
of early brain development in the first three years of life. Includes
excellent short videos on how the brain develops.
Website: developingchild.harvard.edu/science/key-concepts/
brain-architecture

NCAST programs

Provides research-based resources and skills for professionals working with parents of children in the first years of life. The focus is to ensure that young children have nurturing environments. NCAST programs are used extensively at Tresillian to inform nursing practice, most particularly 'Keys to Caregiving' and 'Parent–Child Interaction Scales'.
Website: ncast.org

Crying and prevention of Shaken Baby Syndrome

Period of PURPLE Crying

Provides information and short videos to help you understand why your baby cries, how to soothe her, what Shaken Baby Syndrome is, sleep and self-care.
Website: purplecrying.info

Shaken Baby

Run by Kids Health at The Children's Hospital, Westmead, NSW. There is a video to watch and resources in a range of languages, including Arabic, Dinka, Japanese, Spanish, Cantonese, Farsi, Mandarin, Turkish, Dari, Hindi, Sudanese and Vietnamese.
Website: kidshealth.schn.health.nsw.gov.au/shaken-baby

Multiple birth families

Australian Multiple Birth Association (AMBA)

Enjoy a wide range of online resources, books, DVDs, online forums and clubs to support multiple birth families.
Website: amba.org.au

Your child's health

The Sydney Children's Hospitals Network
Find numbers for emergency services and up-to-date health-info fact sheets listed in alphabetical order.
Website: schn.health.nsw.gov.au/parents-and-carers/find-a-service/
    emergency-services

The Royal Children's Hospital Melbourne
Access up-to-date health-info fact sheets, listed in alphabetical order, covering colic, gastro-oesophageal reflux, fever and many other illnesses. An app is also available with the same information.
Website: rch.org.au/kidsinfo

Raising Children Network: The Australian Parenting Website
Discover a wide range of research-based resources for parents, covering hundreds of topics about raising children from birth through to teenage years.
Website: raisingchildren.net.au

Kidsafe
Learn how to keep your baby safe at home.
Website: kidsafensw.org

Red Nose – saving little lives
Learn from the latest evidence on sleeping your baby safely, how to wrap your baby, how to create a safe sleep environment and what a safe lifestyle looks like.
Website: rednose.com.au/article/archive/C3

Mental health services and resources

PANDA – Perinatal Anxiety & Depression Australia

Discover a range of programs, including a national helpline to support women, men and their families recover from perinatal depression and anxiety.

Website: panda.org.au

PANDA National Helpline: 1300 726 306

    (Mon–Fri, 9 am to 7:30 pm AEST)

Beyond Blue

Focuses specifically on depression and anxiety for men and women. It discusses the cause, treatment and prevention.

Website: beyondblue.org.au

Lifeline

A 24-hour, 7-day-a-week crisis line and suicide prevention service.

Website: lifeline.org.au

Lifeline: 13 11 14 (24 hours a day, 7 days a week)

The Black Dog Institute

Helps both men and women learn about mental illness, including antenatal and postnatal depression and anxiety. It discusses the cause, treatment and prevention of mental illness.

Website: blackdoginstitute.org.au/mental-health-wellbeing/depression

Relationships Australia

Access services and online information focused on improving relationships.

Website: relationships.org.au

Phone contact: 1300 364 277

Gidget Foundation

Resources and support services for families suffering emotional distress during pregnancy and the early parenting period.

Website: gidgetfoundation.com.au

MensLine Australia

Telephone and online counselling services for men's relationship concerns.

Website: mensline.org.au

Phone contact: 1300 78 99 78

Ready to Cope

Sign up for free emails to support you emotionally throughout pregnancy and early motherhood.

Website: cope.org.au/readytocope

COPE – Centre of Perinatal Excellence

Be supported by a range of practical parenting information.

Website: cope.org.au

References

Anders, T., Halpern, L., & Hua, J. (1992). Sleeping Through the Night: A Developmental Perspective. *Pediatrics, 90*(4), 554–560.

Ball, H. (2007). Together or Apart? A Behavioural and Physiological Investigation of Sleeping Arrangements for Twin Babies. *Midwifery, 23*, 404–414. doi:10.1016/j.midw.2006.07.004

Barnard, K. E., Bee, H. L., & Hammond, M. A. (1984). Developmental Changes in Maternal Interactions with Term and Preterm Infants. *Infant Behaviour and Development, 7*, 101–113.

Barr, R., Fairbrother, N., Pauwels, J., Green, J., Chen, M., & Brant, R. (2014). Maternal Frustration, Emotional and Behavioural Responses to Prolonged Infant Crying. *Infant Behaviour and Development, 37*, 652–664. doi:10.1016/j.infbeh.2014.08.012

Belanger, M.-E., Bernier, A., Simard, V., Bordeleau, S., & Carrier, J. (2015). Attachment and Sleep Among Toddlers: Disentangling Attachment Security and Dependency. *Monographs of the Society for Research in Child Development, 80*(1), 125–140. doi:10.1111/mono.12148

Bernier, A., Belanger, M.-E., Tarabulsy, G., Simard, V., & Carrier, J. (2014). My Mother Is Sensitive, But I'm Too Tired to Know: Infant Sleep as a Moderator of Prospective Relations Between Maternal Sensitivity and Infant Outcomes. *Infant Behaviour and Development, 37*, 682–694. doi:10.1016/j.infbeh.2014.08.011

Blunden, S., Thompson, K., & Dawson, D. (2011). Behavioural Sleep Treatments and Night Time Crying in Infants: Challenging the Status Quo. *Sleep Medicine Reviews, 15*, 327–334. doi:10.1016/j.smrv.2010.11.002

Bossi, A., & Hopker, J. (2017). Twilight: Filter the Blue Light of Your Device and Sleep Better. [30.7.17]. *British Journal of Sports Medicine, 51*, 1103–1104. doi:10.1136/bjsports-2016-096315

Brockmann, P., Diaz, B., Damiani, F., Villarroel, L., Nunez, F., & Bruni, O. (2016). Impact of Television on the Quality of Sleep in Preschool Children. *Sleep Medicine, 20*, 140–144. doi:10.1016/j.sleep.2015.06.005

Burnham, M. (2007). The Ontogeny of Diurnal Rhythmicity in Bed-sharing and Solitary-sleeping Infants: A Preliminary Report. *Infant and Child Development, 16*, 341–357. doi:10.1002/icd.520

Countermine, M. S., & Teti, D. M. (2010). Sleep Arrangements and Maternal Adaptation in Infancy. *Infant Mental Health Journal, 31*(6), 647–663. doi:10.1002/imhj.20276

Crncec, R., Cooper, E., & Matthey, S. (2010). Treating Infant Sleep Disturbance: Does Maternal Mood Impact upon Effectiveness? *Journal of Paediatrics and Child Health, 46*, 29–34. doi:10.1111/j.1440.1754.2009.01613.x

Dahlen, H., Foster, J., Psaila, K., Spence, K., Badawi, N., Fowler, C., Schmied, V., & Thornton, C. (2018). Gastro-oesophageal Reflux: A Mixed Methods Study of Infants Admitted to Hospital in the First 12 Months Following Birth in NSW (2000–2011).(Clinical report). *BMC Pediatrics, 18*(1), 1–15. doi:10.1186/s12887-018-0999-9

Davis, K. F., Parker, K., & Montgomery, G. (2004). Sleep in Infants and Young Children: Part One: Normal Sleep. *Journal Pediatric Health Care, 18*, 65–71.

Davis, L., Edwards, H., & Mohay, H. (2003). Mother–Infant Interaction in Premature Infants at Three Months After Nursery Discharge. *International Journal of Nursing Practice, 9*(6), 374–381.

de Graag, J., Cox, R., Hasselman, F., Jansen, J., & de Weerth, C. (2012). Functioning Within a Relationship: Mother–Infant Synchrony and Infant Sleep. *Infant Behaviour and Development, 35*(2) 252–263. doi:10.1016/j.infbeh.2011.12.006

De Marcas, G. S., Soffer-Dudek, N., Dollberg, S., Bar-Haim, Y., & Sadeh, A. (2015). Reactivity and Sleep in Infants: A Longitudinal Objective Assessment. *Monographs of the Society for Research in Child Development, 80*(1), 49–69.

El-Sheikh, M., & Sadeh, A. (2015). Sleep and Development: Introduction to the Monograph. *Monographs of the Society for Research in Child Development, 80*(1), 1–14.

Hayward, K., Johnston, C., Campbell-Yeo, M., Price, S., Houk, S., Whyte, R., White, S., & Caddell, K. (2015). Effect of Cobedding Twins on Coregulation, Infant State, and Twin Safety. *Journal of Obstetric, Gynecologic & Neonatal Nursing, 44*(2), 193–202. doi:10.1111/1552-6909.12557

Health, O. o. K. a. F. N. (2016). *Infants and Children: Acute Management of the Unsettled and Crying Infant.* Sydney NSW: NSW Government Health

Henderson, J., France, K., & Blampied, N. (2011). The Consolidation of Infants' Nocturnal Sleep Across the First Year of Life. *Sleep Medicine Reviews, 15*, 211–220. doi:10.1016/j.smrv.2010.08.003

Henderson, J., Motoi, G., & Blampied, N. (2013). Sleeping Through the Night: A Community Survey of Parents' Opinions About and Expectations of Infant Sleep Consolidation. *Journal of Paediatrics and Child Health, 49*, 535–540. doi:10.1111/jpc.12278

Higley, E., & Dozier, M. (2009). Nighttime Maternal Responsiveness and Infant Attachment at One Year. *Attachment & Human Development, 11*(4), 347–363. doi:10.1080/14616730903016979

Honaker, S., & Meltzer, L. (2014). Bedtime Problems and Night Wakings in Young Children: An Update of the Evidence. *Paediatric Respiratory Reviews, 15*, 333–339. doi:10.1016/j.prrv.2014.04.011

Jian, N., & Teti, D. (2016). Emotional Availability at Bedtime, Infant Temperament, and Infant Sleep Development from One to Six Months. *Sleep Medicine, 23*, 49–58. doi:10.1016/j.sleep.07.001

Kaley, F., Reid, V., & Flynn, E. (2011). The Psychology of Infant Colic: A Review of Current Research. *Infant Mental Health Journal, 32*(5), 526–541. doi:10.1002/imhj.20308

Kaneshi, Y., Ohta, H., Morioka, K., Hayasaka, I., Uzuki, Y., Akimoto, T., … Minakami, H. (2016). Influence of Light Exposure at Nighttime on Sleep Development on Body Growth of Preterm Infants. *Scientific Reports, 6*(21680), 1–8. Retrieved from http://www.nature.com/scientificreports website. doi:10.1038/srep21680

Keefe, M. R., Kotzer, A., Reuss, J., & Sander, L. (1989). Development of a System for Monitoring Infant State Behaviour. *Nursing Research, 38*(6), 344–347.

Kushnir, J., & Sadeh, A. (2011). Sleep of Preschool Children with Night-time Fears. *Sleep Medicine, 12*, 870–874. doi:10.1016/j.sleep.2011.03.022

Laurent, H., & Ablow, J. (2012). The Missing Link: Mothers' Neural Response to Infant Cry Related to Infant Attachment Behaviours. *Infant Behaviour and Development, 35*(4), 761–772. doi:10.1016/j.infbeh.2012.07.007

McCluskey, U., & Duerden, S. (1993). Pre-verbal Communication: The Role of Play in Establishing Rhythms of Communication Between Self and Other. *Journal of Social Work Practice, 7*(1), 17–27. doi:10.1080/02650539308413505

McGraw, K., Hoffmann, R., Harker, C., & Herman, J. (1999). The Development of Circadian Rhythms in a Human Infant. *Sleep, 22*(3), 303–310.

Middlemiss, W. (2004). Defining Problematic Infant Sleep: Shifting the Focus from Deviance to Difference. *Zero to Three, 24*(4), 46–51.

Middlemiss, W., Granger, D. A., Goldberg, W. A., & Nathans, L. (2012). Asynchrony of Mother–Infant Hypothalamic-pituitary-adrenal Axis Activity Following Extinction of Infant Crying Responses Induced During Transition to Sleep. *Early Human Development, 88,* 227–232. doi:10.1016/j.earlhumdev.2011.08.010

Mindell, J. A. (2012). Talking About Babies, Toddlers and Sleep. *Zero to Three, 32*(3), 58–62.

Morrell, J., & Steele, H. (2003). The Role of Attachment Security Temperament, Maternal Perception and Caregiving Behaviour in Persistent Infant Sleeping Problems. *Infant Mental Health Journal, 24*(5), 447–468. doi:10.1002/imhj.10072

Nyquist, K., & Lutes, L. (1998). Co-bedding Twins: A Developmentally Supportive Care Strategy. *Journal of Obstetric, Gynecologic & Neonatal Nursing, 27*(4), 450–456.

Papousek, H., & Papousek, M. (1983). Biological Basis of Social Interactions: Implications of Research for and Understanding of Behavioural Deviance. *Journal of Child Psychology and Psychiatry, 24*(1), 117–129.

Papousek, H., & Papousek, M. (1992). Beyond Emotional Bonding: The Role of Preverbal Communication in Mental Growth and Health. *Infant Mental Health Journal, 13*(1), 43–53.

Peirano, P., Algarin, C., & Uauy, R. (2003). Sleep–Wake States and Their Regulatory Mechanisms Throughout Early Human Development. *The Journal of Pediatrics, 143,* S70–S79.

Pennestri, M.-H., Moss, E., O'Donnell, K., Lecompte, V., Bouvette-Toucot, A.-A., Atkinson, L., . . . Gaudreau, H. (2015). Establishment and Consolidation of the Sleep–Wake Cycle as a Function of Attachment Pattern. *Attachment & Human Development, 17*(1), 23–42. doi:10.1080/14616734.2014.953963

Rivkees, S. A. (2003). Developing Circadian Rhythmicity in Infants. *Pediatrics, 112*(2), 373–381.

Sadeh, A. (2015). Sleep Assessment Methods. *Monographs of the Society for Research in Child Development, 80*(1), 33–48.

Sadeh, A., & Anders, T. (1993). Infant Sleep Problems: Origins, Assessment, Interventions. *Infant Mental Health Journal, 14*(1), 17–34.

Sadeh, A., Mindell, J. A., Luedtke, K., & Wiegand, B. (2009). Sleep and Sleep Ecology in the First 3 Years: A Web-based Study. *Journal Sleep Research, 18*, 60–73. doi:10.1111/j.1365-2869.2008.00699.x

Sadeh, A., Mindell, J. A., & Owens, J. (2011). Why Care About Sleep of Infants and Their Parents. *Sleep Medicine Reviews, 15*, 335–337.

Sadeh, A., Tikotzky, L., & Scher, A. (2010). Parenting and Infant Sleep. *Sleep Medicine Reviews, 14*, 89–96. doi:10.1016/j.smrv.2009.05.003

Scher, A. (2008). Maternal Separation Anxiety as a Regulator of Infants' Sleep. *The Journal of Child Psychology and Psychiatry, 49*(6), 618–625. doi:10.1111/j.1469-7610.2007.01872.x

Scher, A., & Cohen, D. (2015). Sleep as a Mirror of Developmental Transitions in Infancy: The Case of Crawling. *Monographs of the Society for Research in Child Development, 80*(1), 70–88.

Simard, V., Bernier, A., Belanger, M.-E., & Carrier, J. (2013). Infant Attachment and Toddlers' Sleep Assessed by Maternal Reports and Actigraphy: Different Measurement Methods Yield Different Relations. *Journal of Pediatric Psychology, 38*(5), 473–483. doi:10.1093/jpepsy/jst001

Simard, V., Chevalier, V., & Bedard, M.-M. (2017). Sleep and Attachment in Early Childhood: A Series of Meta-analysis. *Attachment & Human Development, 19*(3), 298–321. doi:10.1080/146 16734.2017.1293703

Sinclair, D., Staton, S., Smith, S., Pattinson, C., Marriott, A., & Thorpe, K. (2016). What Parents Want: Parent Preference Regarding Sleep for Their Preschool Child When Attending Early Care and Education. *Sleep Health, 2*, 12–18. doi:10.1016/j. sleh.2015.11.002

Soltis, J. (2004). The Signal Functions of Infant Crying. *Behavioural and Brain Sciences, 27*(4), 443–490.

Spietz, A., Johnson-Crowley, N., Sumner, G., & Barnard, K. (2008). *Keys to Caregiving*. University Washington, Seattle, Washington USA: NCAST Programs.

St James-Roberts, I., & Peachey, E. (2011). Distinguishing Infant Prolonged Crying from Sleep-waking Problems. *Archives of Disease in Childhood, 96*(4), 340–344. doi:10.1136/adc.2010.200204

St James-Roberts, I., Roberts, M., Hovish, K., & Owen, C. (2016). Descriptive Figures for Differences in Parenting and Infant Night-time Distress in the First Three Months of Age. *Primary Health Care Research & Development, 17*, 611–621. doi:10.1017/ S1463423616000293

Staton, S., Marriott, A., Pattinson, C., Smith, S., Sinclair, D., & Thorpe, K. (2016). Supporting Sleep in Early Care and Education: An Assessment of Observed Sleep Times Using a Sleep Practices Optimality Index. *Sleep Health, 2*, 30–34. doi:10.1016/j. sleh.2015.12.005

Stern, D. (2000). The Sense of Core Self: II. Self with Other. *The Interpersonal World of the Infant* (1st Paperback ed., pp. 100–123). New York, USA: Basic Books. (Reprinted from: 2000).

Stern, D. (2002). The Infant's Repertoire. *The First Relationship* (2nd ed., pp. 49–68). London, England: Harvard University Press. (Reprinted from: 2002).

Stockton, D. (2007). Caring for Twins. *Practical Parenting*, May 2007, 78–81.

Teng, A., Bartle, A., Sadeh, A., & Mindell, J. A. (2012). Infant and Toddler Sleep in Australia and New Zealand. *Journal of Paediatrics and Child Health, 48*, 268–273. doi:10.1111/j.1440-1754.2011.02251.x

Thoman, E. (1990). Sleeping and Waking States in Infants: A Functional Perspective. *Neuroscience & Biobehavioural Reviews, 14*, 93–107.

Thomas, K. A., Burr, R., Spieker, S., Lee, J., & Chen, J. (2014). Mother–Infant Circadian Rhythm: Development of Individual Patterns and Dyadic Synchrony. *Early Human Development, 90*, 885–890. doi:10.1016/j.earlhumdev.214.09.005

Tikotzky, L., & Sadeh, A. (2009). Maternal Sleep-related Cognitions and Infant Sleep: A Longitudinal Study from Pregnancy through the First Year. *Child Development, 80*(3), 860–874.

Tikotzky, L., Sadeh, A., Volkovich, E., Manber, R., Meiri, G., & Shahar, G. (2015). Infant Sleep Development from 3 to 6 Months Postpartum: Links with Maternal Sleep and Paternal Involvement. *Monographs of the Society for Research in Child Development, 80*, 107–124.

Tsai, S., Barnard, K. E., Lentz, M. J., & Thomas, K. A. (2011). Mother–Infant Activity Synchrony as a Correlate of the Emergence of Circadian Rhythm. *Biological Research for Nursing, 13*(1), 80–88. doi:10.1177/1099800410378889

Tsai, S., Thomas, K. A., Lentz, M. J., & Barnard, K. E. (2012). Light Is Beneficial for Infant Circadian Entrainment: An Actigraphic Study.

Journal of Advanced Nursing, 68(8), 1738–1747. doi:10.1111/j.1365-2648.2011.05857.x

Vaughn, B., El-Sheikh, M., Shin, N., Elmore-Staton, L., Krzysik, L., & Monteiro, L. (2011). Attachment Representations, Sleep Quality and Adaptive Functioning in Preschool Children. *Attachment & Human Development, 13*(6), 525–540. doi:10.1080/14616734.2011.608984

Volling, B., McElwain, N., & Miller, A. (2002). Emotion Regulation in Context: The Jealousy Complex between Young Siblings and Its Relations with Child and Family Characteristics. *Child Development, 73*(2), 581–600.

Yale, M., Messinger, D., Cobo-Lewis, A., & Delgado, C. (2003). The Temporal Coordination of Early Infant Communication. *Developmental Psychology, 39*(5), 815–824. doi:10.1037/0012-1649.39.5.815

Index

soothing, failure in 93–4, 110
3 months, after 107
what you can do 101–2, 109–10

daily rhythms, external 11–19
day-night rhythm, establishing 7–10,
    11–12, 22
  daylight 7
  feeding and socialising 13–14
daytime routine, establishing 12–13, 22

ear infections 272

feeding, socialising and activity
    patterns 11–13, 27
  daytime feeding 13–14
  night feeds 14–15
fevers 270–1, 274

gastro-oesophageal reflux (GOR) 257–8
gastro-oesophageal reflux disease
    (GORD) 258–9

hands-on settling technique 153
holidays 80–5, 87
  establishing routines 83–5
  jet lag management 83

infant colic 252–4, 274
  calming techniques 255
  possible remedies 254–6

light, role in sleep 5–6, 10, 22, 221
  blue light 6, 9, 50, 79, 218, 219
  smartphones, tablets and TVs 6, 79,
    218–19

melatonin 6–10, 30
  breastmilk 8
multiple births see twins and sleep

night terrors 264–5
  indicators of 264
  managing 265
night-time fears 261–3, 274
  anxieties about personal situations,
    managing 263

darkness and monsters fears,
    managing 262
nightmares 260–1

parental presence settling technique
    172, 180
playtime 17–19
pram, selecting 15
preschoolers (3 to 5 years) 201–3, 224
  caffeine 217
  calming bedtime routine 210–11
  daytime napping 217
  emotion management, helping 205–8
  inconsistent bedtimes 218
  limit-setting for sleep 213–15
  playing in bed 216
routines and sleep needs 208–9
  sleep environment 221–2
  sleep problems 212–22
  social-emotional world 204–8
  stalling/refusal to go to bed 213–15
  stimulating activities and sleep 216
  strategies for handling bedtime
    stalling 215
  strategies for settling 220
  trouble falling asleep/staying asleep
    215–19
  TVs, video games, computers, tablets
    and smartphones 218–19

'quiet sleep' 26–9

reflux 257–9
resources 275–82
Responsive Settling 142–3, 170–3
  comfort settling technique 171
  hands-on settling technique 153
  parental presence settling technique
    172
  putting baby to bed awake 170–3
  soothing-in-arms technique 143

safety measures for head banging,
    rocking and rolling 266
self-settling 33, 37–8, 44, 59, 62, 151–2
  active soothing by parent instead of
    49–50